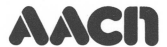

Standards
for
Nursing Care
of the
Critically Ill

AMERICAN ASSOCIATION OF CRITICAL-CARE NURSES

STANDARDS FOR NURSING CARE OF THE CRITICALLY ILL

AACn

STANDARDS FOR NURSING CARE OF THE CRITICALLY ILL

Edited by AACN Standards Committee:

Judith Thierer, RN
Co-Chairperson

Susan Perhus, RN, BSN, CCRN

M. Lynn McCracken, RN, MS

Margaret A. Reynolds, RN, MSN

Aline M. Holmes, RN, MSN, CCRN
Co-Chairperson

Barbara Turton, RN, BSN

Deborah Swanson Berkowitz, RN

Joanne M. Disch, RN, MSN, CCRN

Reston Publishing Company, Inc.
A Prentice-Hall Company
Reston, Virginia

Developed by the American Association of Critical-Care Nurses. Funded in part by the Health Resources Administration, Division of Nursing—Grant No. D10 NU 29018.

These Standards represent the philosophy of the American Association of Critical-Care Nurses and are statements of quality which serve as a model for care of the critically ill; they do not constitute a legal or regulatory obligation to a patient.

The AACN Standards are endorsed by the Society of Critical Care Medicine.

Library of Congress Cataloging in Publication Data

American Association of Critical-Care Nurses.
  Standards for nursing care of the critically ill.

  1. Intensive care nursing—Standards. 2. Intensive care units—Standards. I. Thierer, Judith.
II. Holmes, Aline M. III. American Association of
Critical-Care Nurses. Standards Committee. IV. Title.
[DNLM: 1. Critical care—Standards—Nursing texts.
WY 154 S7854]
RT120.I5A43 1980b   610.73′61   80-24387
ISBN 0-8359-7061-2

10 9 8 7 6 5 4 3 2

Printed in the United States of America

American Association of Critical-Care Nurses
P.O. Box C-19528, Irvine, California 92713
2192 Martin Drive, Suite 200, Irvine, California 92715
(714) 752-8191

CONTENTS

PREFACE

The editors encourage readers to examine this document with emphasis on the utilization of the Standards. While the examples of implementation are provided for illustrative purposes to aid the reader in exploring possible methods of utilization, they do not represent complete case studies, nor are they designed to provide chronological sequencing.

At times, nursing actions illustrated in the document may appear to be made independently without collaboration from administration and/or physicians. It should be noted, however, that in these instances, an assumption has been made, but not explicitly stated, that when needed, appropriate collaboration has occurred and interventions are in conformance with administrative policies.

Field testing participants stressed that a thorough understanding of the intended utilization of the document (Part I-B, Implementation) prior to studying the standards themselves was beneficial. This permits the reader full comprehension of the impact of these standards upon nursing practice, the environment, and the care of the critically ill patient.

ACKNOWLEDGMENTS

Associations such as AACN accomplish their activities through the efforts of dedicated members who give of their time and energy. Nowhere in the history of the Association has this been better exemplified than by the members of the Standards Committee. These individuals have demonstrated a commitment to the quality of care delivered to the critically ill that has carried them through four years of intensive effort. The synergism of this group has been described by each as an exceptional professional experience and has produced a product that is certainly greater than the sum of its parts. While there is no way to compensate Association volunteers for their contributions, the committee's reward will be realized when utilization of the Standards results in improved care for the critically ill.

The Committee wishes to recognize especially the contributions of two deceased committee members, Mary Jo O'Brien and Marion Reichle. Both Mary Jo and Marion were involved in the committee's initial activities and were instrumental in directing the group's efforts toward a comprehensive and clinically relevant document. It is difficult to identify all the people whose ideas and expertise have contributed to a project of this magnitude. The Committee recognizes the contributions of those individuals with whom we have interacted in our nursing careers, and who have influenced our attitudes toward critical care nursing. More specifically, the committee wishes to acknowledge those critical care nursing leaders and experts in related areas who contributed directly to the content of this document. Those individuals who contributed to the Process Standards are Karen Anderson, Charold Baer, Pamela McCullough, Nancy Molter and Marilyn Ricci. Those who contributed to the Structure Standards are Robert Benedetti, Helen Benedikter, William Betts, Donald Billie, Max Brown, Kathleen DeLuca, Carolyn Ehrlich, Paula Fleurant, Rita Froelich, Eddie Hedrick, Marguerite Kinney, Norma Lang, A. D. Lewis, Carol Lindeman, Louise Mansfield, Ida Martinson, Annalee Oakes, Charles Rice, John Ryan and John Swope. The committee is especially pleased and proud to have had Norma Lang as a consultant in the development of this document. All of these individuals gave generously of their time and expertise to enhance the quality of care delivered to the critically ill.

Field testing to assure clinical relevance and readability was conducted prior to publication of this document. Four hospitals and one AACN Chapter were selected as sites for the field test. The hospitals involved were De Paul Hospital, Cheyenne, Wyoming; Barnes Hospital, St. Louis, Missouri; Holyoke Hospital, Holyoke, Massachusetts; and Morton F. Plant Hospital, Clearwater, Florida. The AACN Chapter involved was the Upper East

Tennessee Chapter. The individuals who participated in this process provided thoughtful and constructive comments which enhanced the quality of the document, and the committee is grateful for the enthusiasm and commitment demonstrated by each participant.

AACN staff members Linda Simpson (1975–1977) and Mary Jane Bromley (1978–1979), provided staff support for the committee's activities. AACN national office administrative staff members Nancy Gibson and Virginia Real are recognized for their efforts in the development of this document.

Judith Thierer, RN
Co-Chairperson, Standards
Committee

STANDARDS FOR
NURSING CARE
OF THE
CRITICALLY ILL

DEVELOPMENT
OF
STANDARDS

Part I-A

EVOLUTION AND PHILOSOPHY

Accountability is a significant characteristic and responsibility of every profession. Historically, many have questioned nursing's right to be called a profession, perhaps rightly so. Nursing has traditionally functioned in a delegatory role which did not invite accountability. In the process of professional development, nursing has expanded its body of knowledge, increased its interest and participation in research, addressed role delineation, and accepted accountability. The need to define quality in nursing care and to evaluate the quality of its delivery has been a natural outcome of this professional growth process. Additionally, extrinsic societal forces now manifest an "era of accountability" emphasizing the need for nursing to accept the challenge of fulfilling its professional responsibilities.

Development of *Standards for Nursing Care of the Critically Ill* has been one of the goals of the American Association of Critical-Care Nurses (AACN) since the Association's inception in 1969. AACN's first five years of evolution were concerned with other priorities such as educational programming, a national office organization, development of the *Core Curriculum for Critical-Care Nursing*, and the certification examination. During 1974, when the external and internal climate of nursing reflected a growing interest in quality assurance, AACN cooperated with the American Nurses' Association's (ANA) task force which developed "Guidelines for Review of Nursing Care at the Local Level." Thereafter, an AACN committee was formed and charged with the task of developing "Standards."

The Committee's initial search of current literature revealed diverse opinions among nursing leaders concerning the appropriateness and efficacy of various methods of evaluating health care delivery. In addition, quality assurance terminology was confusing. Some authors used "standards" when referring to a set of patient outcomes, others described "standards" as a numerical level of performance, and still others used "standards" to identify those restrictions and/or guidelines imposed by regulatory agencies. The Committee also examined standards previously developed by other authors and associations. While substantial accomplishments were evident, standards which could be readily implemented by the practicing critical care nurse were nonexistent.

Based upon the results of the Committee's initial activities and their collective clinical experiences, the Standards Committee concluded that no single approach to evaluation was sufficient. Rather, multiple approaches would be necessary to provide a comprehensive evaluation program. The Committee further concluded that every effort would be made to use existing terminology rather than a jargon particular only to its document and

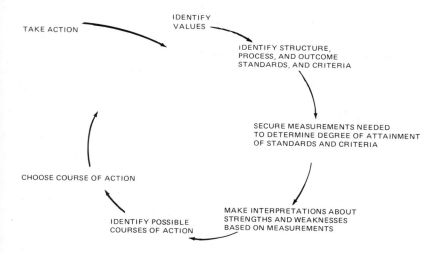

IDENTIFY VALUES

TAKE ACTION

IDENTIFY STRUCTURE, PROCESS, AND OUTCOME STANDARDS, AND CRITERIA

SECURE MEASUREMENTS NEEDED TO DETERMINE DEGREE OF ATTAINMENT OF STANDARDS AND CRITERIA

CHOOSE COURSE OF ACTION

MAKE INTERPRETATIONS ABOUT STRENGTHS AND WEAKNESSES BASED ON MEASUREMENTS

IDENTIFY POSSIBLE COURSES OF ACTION

Adapted from Lang, Norma, "A Model for Quality Assurance in Nursing," 1974, with participation.

Figure 1. Model for Quality Assurance: Implementation of Standards. (Copyright 1975 by the American Nurses Association. Reprinted with permission.)

to build upon the efforts of others. Therefore, similarities exist between AACN's Process Standards and ANA's Standards of Practice, since both are based upon the nursing process as the fundamental method for delivery of nursing care.

Development of this document corresponds to the initial steps of Lang's quality assurance model, depicted in Figure 1. The Association's values were identified by reviewing the purposes of the Association as well as AACN's philosophy and definition of critical care nursing practice. The philosophy of the American Association of Critical-Care Nurses states that "each critically ill person has the right to expect nursing care provided by a critical care nurse." Critical care nursing practice is defined as

the utilization of the nursing process in the prevention of and intervention in life-threatening situations. This practice shall be based on:

(a) a thorough knowledge of the interrelatedness of body systems and the dynamic nature of the life process;

(b) a recognition and appreciation of the individual's wholeness, uniqueness, and significant social and environmental relationships;

(c) an appreciation of the importance of the collaborative role of all members of the health team.

Integral components of this practice are:

(a) individual professional accountability;

(b) the pursuit of knowledge and clinical expertise through continuing education.

Subsequent steps of the model involve implementation of the standards. Methods of implementation are addressed in Part I–B, Implementation of Standards.

The Committee does not perceive the Standards as a static, completed document. Just as the quality assurance model is open and circular to indicate its dynamic nature, the Standards are viewed as a working document, subject to the modification and revision necessitated by the dynamic nature of critical care nursing.

BIBLIOGRAPHY

American Nurses' Association, *A Plan for Implementation of the Standards of Nursing Practice*, Kansas City, Mo.: ANA, 1975.

Cantor, Marjorie M., *Achieving Nursing Care Standards*, Wakefield, Mass.: Internal and External Nursing Resources, Inc., 1978.

Lang, Norma M., "Are Professional Nurses Ready for Quality Assurance Program," Journal New York State Nurses' Association, 5:24–32, November, 1975.

Nicholls, M. E. and V. G. Wessels, *Nursing Standards and Nursing Process*, Wakefield, Mass.: Contemporary Publishing, Inc., 1978.

Critical care nursing practice is a dynamic process, the scope of which is defined in terms of the critically ill patient, the critical care nurse and the environment in which critical care nursing is delivered; all three components are essential elements for the practice of critical care nursing.

SCOPE OF CRITICAL CARE NURSING PRACTICE

The Critically Ill Patient

The critically ill patient is characterized by the presence of real or potential life-threatening health problems and by the requirement for continuous observation and intervention to prevent complications and restore health. The concept of the critically ill patient includes the patient's family and/or significant others.

The Critical Care Nurse

The critical care nurse is a registered professional nurse committed to ensuring that all critically ill patients receive optimal care. This nurse's practice is based on the following:

1. Individual professional accountability

2. Thorough knowledge of the interrelatedness of body systems and the dynamic nature of the life process

3. Recognition and appreciation of the individual's wholeness, uniqueness and significant social and environmental relationships

4. Appreciation of the collaborative role of all members of the health care team

To continually refine the practice, the critical care nurse participates in ongoing educational activities. In addition to basic preparation, the critical care nurse acquires an advanced knowledge of psychosocial, physiological and therapeutic components specific to the care of the critically ill. Clinical competency and the ability to effectively interact with patients, families and other members of the health care team are developed. Additionally, an awareness of the nurse's responsibility for a therapeutic environment is cultivated.

The critical care nurse utilizes the nursing process as a framework for practice. In caring for the critically ill, the nurse will collect data, identify and determine the priority of the patient's problems/needs, formulate an appropriate plan of nursing care, implement the plan of nursing care according to the priority of the identified problems/needs, and evaluate the process and outcome of nursing care.

The Critical Care Environment

A critical care unit is any geographically designated area which is designed to facilitate the care of the critically ill patient by critical care nurses. It is an area where safety, organizational and ethical standards are maintained for patient welfare. Although critical care nursing usually occurs in a critical care unit, it can occur in any setting that meets the environmental and nursing standards such as an area which has a psychologically supportive environment for patients and significant others, adequately functioning equipment and supplies, readily available emergency equipment, facilities to meet staff needs, and ready access to support departments.

This Scope of Practice statement provides a definition and framework for nursing care of the critically ill. For critical care nursing practice to occur, all three components must be present: the critically ill patient, the critical care nurse and a therapeutic critical care environment. The *Standards for Nursing Care of the Critically Ill* are viewed as an extension of the Scope of Practice and offer more specific guidance to nurses delivering care to the critically ill.

CRITICAL CARE NURSE: See "Scope of Practice" statement, page 5.

CRITICAL CARE UNIT: See "Scope of Practice" statement, page 5.

CRITICALLY ILL PATIENT: See "Scope of Practice" statement, page 5.

GOAL: The desired outcome; the end toward which effort is directed.

NEED: A physiological or psychological requirement for the well being of a human being.

OBJECTIVE DATA: The data that express the use of measurable and observable facts, without distortion by personal feelings, as those facts relate to a specific problem/need.

OUTCOME: The result to be achieved.

PROBLEM: A situation involving an existing or potential difficulty necessitating inquiry, consideration, or solution.

PROCESS: A series of actions, changes, or functions that bring about an end or result.

STANDARD: Standards for care of the critically ill are statements of quality which serve as a model to facilitate and evaluate the delivery of optimal nursing care to the critically ill.

STRUCTURE: The environment within which care is given including organizational and management characteristics, qualifications of health professionals, staffing, physical facilities, and equipment.

SUBJECTIVE DATA: Information regarding the patient's feelings, concerns, description of symptoms; statements from the patient and/or significant others.

TECHNICAL COMPETENCE: The ability to perform psychomotor skills safely by following a specified procedure.

IMPLEMENTATION
OF
STANDARDS

Part I–B

AACN's purpose in developing standards is to improve the quality of care delivered to the critically ill; this can only be achieved, however, through appropriate implementation of the standards. *Standards for Nursing Care of the Critically Ill* provide a means of assessment of the quality of care and a guide for subsequent corrective actions; the crucial test of the standards will be the extent to which these implementation activities occur.

The overall plan for implementation of standards has previously been addressed and is illustrated in Figure 1. More specific plans for implementation may take any of several forms, depending upon the needs and resources of a given nurse and/or agency. In the following sections, approaches to implementation are illustrated. It is anticipated that many other methods of implementation will be identified and utilized by the critical care nursing community.

IMPLEMENTATION BY THE INDIVIDUAL PRACTITIONER

One form of implementing the *Standards for Nursing Care of the Critically Ill* is through individual nurses who view themselves as professional persons, accountable for the quality of care they deliver. Critical care nurses should compare the care they personally deliver with that suggested by the process standards. When a discrepancy exists, the nurse may select alternative actions to improve care. Often, the example accompanying the standard will illustrate actions to be taken, and AACN's *Core Curriculum for Critical-Care Nursing* and other texts will provide sources for review or clarification of concepts. When corrective actions have been implemented, the nurse may then compare again, and continue the cycle.

Structure standards may be implemented in a similar manner. The standards assist the practitioner in identification of those structural or environmental supports which are necessary for care delivery. When comparison indicates a deficiency in the environment, actions can be directed toward correction.

Implicit in the implementation activities suggested for the individual practitioner is the concept of change, and in this respect, the standards should be viewed as an instrument of change. For example, if a nurse encounters a process standard that the nurse consistently neglects in practice, some form of internal change will be necessary and should be reflected in a behavioral change to meet the standard. The needed change may also extend beyond the individual nurse to others in the organization. The nurse might identify a need for an orientation program or a new piece of equipment to achieve specific structure standards; this calls for the involvement of many individuals if the change is to be successful.

Implementation by an agency or group of practitioners can occur either through the formal and permanent structures within the agency, or through the more informal channels and groups that exist. A formal structure that usually has the most potential for successfully implementing standards within an organization is the nursing committee. A hospital nursing service department generally has a committee of this type concerned with the evaluation of practice, identified as the "Nursing Practice Committee," "Nursing Audit Committee," "Standards Committee," or "Quality Assurance Committee." Regardless of its label, the committee should establish the following:

1. Evaluation philosophy and purpose
2. Evaluation policies
3. Evaluation standards
4. Evaluation methodologies
5. Plans for utilization of evaluation findings

One committee only should be responsible for the evaluaton of care delivered by nurses within the setting or agency, rather than having each of several committees focus upon slightly different aspects of evaluation. For purposes of interdisciplinary evaluation, however, a second committee may be warranted, with interaction between the two committees.

As an example, one hospital established a "Nursing Quality Assurance Committee" which was responsible for all ongoing evaluation of nursing care within the institution. The approach to evaluation was based upon the Model for Quality Assurance (Figure 1) and the evaluation standards as stated in the section on structure standards. To utilize the *Standards for Nursing Care of the Critically Ill*, the committee transformed each of the standards into their already existing audit format; the result was an audit tool which was used to conduct both retrospective and concurrent evaluation in all critical care units. After the initial evaluation, the committee identified standards which were not achieved and recommended courses of action which would facilitate standard achievement.

In another setting, a less formal method was used to implement the standards. The head nurse of the coronary care unit secured several copies of *Standards for Nursing Care of the Critically Ill* and asked the staff to review the document carefully. A meeting was held to discuss plans for implementation of the standards; several nurses were assigned the task of evaluating the extent to which their unit met each of the standards. Numerous methods were used to perform the evaluation, including record audit, questionnaire, direct observation of nurses and patients, and di-

IMPLEMENTATION BY AN AGENCY AND/OR GROUP OF PRACTITIONERS

rect examination of policies, procedures, and equipment. Achievements and deficiencies were identified with respect to each of the standards and presented to the entire staff. All personnel participated in developing a plan for corrective action to promote achievement of standards not yet attained. In some instances, large scale organizational change was necessary, while other changes could easily be instituted within the unit. Six months later, the nurses conducted a similar evaluation and revised their plans for corrective action as needed.

Another example of implementation involves using the standards in evaluation of personnel. The head nurses of three critical care units recognized the potential of the standards to provide substance to their personnel evaluations. They invited their supervisors and staff nurse representatives to join them in the task of developing a personnel evaluation form based upon the *Standards for Nursing Care of the Critically Ill*. Through development of this evaluation tool, the nurses were eventually able to define specific levels of practice within each standard, resulting in a clinical ladder for professional advancement in critical care nursing. Nurses seeking advancement were asked to document their ability to implement the standards.

In still another setting, the critical care coordinator and the staff development department collaborated in implementation of the standards. Critical care unit orientees were expected to read the standards in an effort to acquaint them with eventual performance expectations. Throughout the orientation period, the standards were used to guide learning experiences. Each orientee later demonstrated personal implementation of the process standards in a case presentation.

Implementation of the standards by an agency or group of practitioners generally implies more extensive change than does implementation by an individual. Because this type of change is more complex, nurses are encouraged to give careful thought and planning to implementation activities. The few examples previously illustrated may be helpful in generating ideas for implementation, but creative adaptations will be required for each specific setting.

IMPLEMENTATION THROUGH SYSTEMATIC STUDY

An important means of implementing the standards is through systematic study of selected topics. The initial step in this process is review of the standards to identify meaningful topics. Selecting topics of significance to critical care delivery is likely to yield results which will substantially improve the quality of care.

Stating the topic in the form of a question may help to clarify the exact topic and provide direction for systematic study; when the question is clearly stated, measurement is simplified. The following are several examples of study topics:

1. *Infection Control:*   Do nurses in the critical care unit document the signs and symptoms of infection on the health care record? Are interventions for the symptoms appropriate? Are they documented in the record?

2. *Physical Facility Planning:*   What is the average length of time required for a unit of blood to be ordered and received by the unit?

3. *Management:*   What percent of patients admitted to the unit in the past year have had primary medical diagnoses that were included in the admission criteria of the unit?

4. *Process Standards:*

(a) What percentage of patients admitted to the critical care unit in the past three months had evidence in their records of an initial physical assessment performed within twenty-four hours of admission?

(b) What percent of patient records document that the critical care nurse involved the patient and/or significant others in the formulation of goals?

(c) What percent of critical care orientees are able to correctly identify, in writing, standing orders for intervention in acute life-threatening dysrhythmias?

Once a topic has been identified and stated in measurable terms, the study method must be selected. It is important to select the method that will yield the necessary information or answer the study question. A partial list of methods follows:

1. Retrospective record audit
2. Concurrent record audit
3. Direct observation of patients
4. Interview/questionnaire of patients
5. Interview/questionnaire of nurses
6. Direct observation of nurse performance
7. Self-review/evaluation
8. Supervisor review/evaluation
9. Peer review/evaluation
10. Utilization review

11. Direct observation of equipment/facilities
12. Critical incident reports
13. Grand rounds
14. Patient care conferences

Some methods are more useful in measuring a particular topic than others; each method has advantages and disadvantages. For example, the accuracy of information secured from a patient's health record is dependent upon the recording practices of the practitioner who documents in the record. Direct observation is generally considered to yield more accurate information, although it too is subject to inaccuracy and observer bias.

When the topic and study method have been selected, the systematic study can proceed. One of the study topics mentioned previously can serve again as an illustration

> What percentage of patients admitted to the critical care unit in the past three months had evidence in their records of an initial physical assessment performed within twenty-four hours of admission?

In most units, the volume of patients admitted during a three month period is too large to allow examination of all records for evidence of physical assessment. The total number of records could be reduced to a more manageable number by any of several means. A random sample of perhaps twenty-five records could be selected from the total and reviewed for evidence of the standard; or the study population could be narrowed according to specific characteristics. Perhaps only the records of patients thirty-forty years old would be reviewed, or review would be limited to those patients with specific diagnoses. Once the method is decided, the records would be retrieved from the patient record department and systematically examined for evidence of physical assessments within twenty-four hours after admission. Decisions for subsequent actions would be based upon the findings.

IMPLEMENTATION IN CONJUNCTION WITH OTHER STANDARDS

The *Standards for Nursing Care of the Critically Ill* reflect a generic or general approach to evaluation and are not specific to patient populations or settings. Therefore, nurses are encouraged to use the AACN Standards in conjunction with standards available from other sources. For example, the Process Standards call for various kinds of data when assessing any critically ill patient. The nurse assessing a critically ill patient with cardiovascular problems may also want to use ANA's Standards of Cardiovascular Nursing Practice to identify the assessment factors specific to the cardiovascular patient. As another example, nurses should identify and use appropriate state fire and safety codes in conjunction with the AACN *Standards*, since state codes are generally more specific to the region or locale; such codes are legal requirements, as well.

A number of nursing organizations, state and national agencies, and accrediting bodies have identified and published standards which may be used in conjunction with the *Standards for Nursing Care of the Critically Ill*. Many of these are listed as follows:

Association of Operating Room Nurses

Emergency Department Nurses Association

Nurses Association of the American College of Obstetricians and Gynecologists

American Association of Nephrology Nurses and Technicians

American Association of Neurosurgical Nurses

Oncology Nursing Society

Orthopedic Nurses Association

American Nurses' Association
  Standards of Nursing Practice
  Standards of Geriatric Nursing Practice
  Standards of Maternal and Child Health Nursing Practice
  Standards of Psychiatric and Mental Health Nursing Practice
  Standards of Community Mental Health Nursing Practice
  Standards of Medical-Surgical Nursing Practice
  Standards of Cardiovascular Nursing Practice
  Standards of Orthopedic Nursing Practice
  Standards of Nursing Practice: Operating Room
  Standards of Emergency Nursing Practice

City, State, and National Codes

Joint Commission on Accreditation of Hospitals

Department of Health and Human Resources

IMPLEMENTATION THROUGH OTHER MECHANISMS

Implementation of the standards impacts every facet of professional activity. Therefore, the significance of assessing the quality of care delivered to the critically ill must pervade the Association's activities just as it should pervade the activities of each critical care practitioner and agency.

Direct methods of utilizing the standards have previously been identified. Other methods exist which are more indirect, but are equally important in achieving implementation. For example, the standards may be incorporated into accreditation mechanisms since the standards provide an objective basis for evaluating an agency's ability to deliver care to the critically ill.

The concept of evaluation which is, in essence, implementation of the standards will be integrated into future AACN activities. The standards will be incorporated into the CCRN certification program. Critical care nurses will be evaluated on their ability to achieve the standards. The standards will provide a basis for the content of educational activities and a sense of direction for long range planning. AACN chapters will serve an essential and pivotal role in facilitating implementation of the standards. Through their membership, chapters will influence both individual practitioners and agencies and will provide feedback to the Association regarding mechanisms and/or problems of implementation.

Because they cross geographical and organizational boundaries, the mechanisms identified above present a broad scope for implementation. They will, therefore, have a profound influence on the future of critical care nursing.

EVALUATION
OF
STANDARDS

Part I-C

It is important to reiterate that the *Standards for Nursing Care of the Critically Ill* is a working document, subject to evaluation and subsequent modification, thus reflecting the dynamic nature of critical care nursing. The American Association of Critical-Care Nurses is anxious to involve its membership in this process of evaluation. All nurses involved in the care of the critically ill are invited to exercise responsibility for evaluation of the standards and to share their feedback with the Association. Numerous mechanisms may be used to provide evaluation feedback, including the following:

Incorporation of the standards into AACN workshops and educational programs with emphasis upon their implementation and evaluation.

Opportunities for informal discussion on the standards at AACN regional workshops.

Solicitation of opinions and problems through *Focus on AACN*.

3M award topic on implementation or evaluation of the standards.

Solicitation of articles discussing implementation and evaluation of the standards for inclusion in *Heart and Lung, The Journal of Critical Care* or *Focus on AACN*.

Availability of AACN professional staff by telephone or mail to receive direct feedback from the membership.

STRUCTURE
STANDARDS

Part II-A

VALUE STATEMENT

The critical care nurse shall be cognizant of and have concern for those factors which ensure a safe and effective environment in which care to the critically ill is delivered.

COMPREHENSIVE STANDARD I: The critical care unit shall be designed to ensure a safe and supportive environment for critically ill patients and for the personnel who care for them.

Supporting Standards	Examples of Implementation	References
The critical care nurse shall participate in the development of the philosophy of use, and in the designing and planning of new or renovated critical care units.	The critical care nurse should actively participate in the functional phase of designing a unit, when the purpose and planned use of the unit are described. Once that has been determined, the design and planning phase can occur, with emphasis on providing a safe and supportive environment in which to give care to the critically ill.	Clipson, C. W., and J. J. Wehrer, Planning for Cardiac Care-A Guide to the Planning and Design of Cardiac Care Facilities. Copyright by the University of Michigan, 1973, The Health Administration Press, M2210 School of Public Health, The University of Michigan, Ann Arbor, Michigan.
The critical care nurse shall be cognizant of various rules and/or regulations governing physical facilities for care of critically ill patients, such as those established by the: —city —state —Department of Health, Education, and Welfare —Joint Commission on Accreditation of Hospitals		Collins, J. A., and W. F. Ballinger, The Surgical Intensive Care Unit, *Surgery*, September, 1969, 614–619. Department of Health, Education, and Welfare, How to Plan and Design Intensive and Coronary Care Units, *Hospital Topics*, October, 1973. (HEW Publication No. HRA 74–4007)
The critical care nurse shall ensure that the patient's privacy is protected without losing constant surveillance capability through the planning and design of the critical care unit.	The critical care nurses at Hospital A were instrumental in designing clear glass sliding doors for patient cubicles with drapes which could be pulled for privacy.	Department of Health, Education, and Welfare, Minimum Requirements of Construction and Equipment for Hospital and Medical Facilities, (HEW Publication No. HRA 76–400).
The critical care nurse shall ensure that the following components are considered in the planning and design of the unit: —adequate space per patient bed, with consideration of potential equipment needs —adequate illumination		Grogan, Sr. M. Hildegard. A Study of the Verbalized Perceptions of Patients to Environmental Quiet Induced by a New Intensive Care Unit Design. Unpublished Master's Dissertation, School of Nursing, Catholic University of America, April, 1972.

Supporting Standards	Examples of Implementation	References

—windows, clocks, calendars
—plumbing/sewage and sinks
—use of proper colors for walls, ceilings, and furnishings
—use of acoustic materials to minimize noise
—life support systems, including medical gases, suction outlets, and emergency power availability
—adequate space for support areas, including but not limited to:
  —nursing station
  —office space
  —clean and soiled utility areas
  —linen storage
  —equipment storage
  —medication room
  —janitor's closet
  —visitors' waiting area
  —conference room
  —staff lounge area
  —nourishment station
  —emergency equipment storage
  —adequate ventilation and humidity/temperature control individualized for each patient room.
		Joint Commission on Accreditation of Hospitals. *Accreditation Manual.* Standards for Special Care Units.
		
		Kinney, J. M., and C. W. Walter, The Design of an Intensive Care Unit, *Manual of Surgical Intensive Care,* ed. J. M. Kinney. Philadelphia: W. B. Saunders Co., 1977.
		
		Kornfeld, D. S., et al. Psychological Hazards of the Intensive Care Unit, *Nursing Clinics of North America,* 3, March, 1968, 41–51.
		
		Skillman, J. J., *Intensive Care.* Boston: Little, Brown and Company, 1975, Chapter 1.
		
		Vaisrub, S., Windows for the Soul, *Archives of Internal Medicine,* 130, August, 1972, 297.

The critical care nurse shall ensure that a communication system within the unit provides for: —routine patient care —notifying appropriate personnel in emergencies		
The critical care nurse shall ensure that the monitoring systems are appropriate to the needs of the patient population.	The critical care nurse working in a respiratory intensive care unit ensures that there is an appropriate system to monitor intrapulmonary pressures, arterial blood gases, etc. On a general medical unit, one of the pulmonary patients developed a pneumothorax and required an arterial line to allow for frequent blood gases. Since	

Supporting Standards	*Examples of Implementation*	*References*
	he was in a single room at the end of the hall, the charge nurse was concerned about the danger to the patient should the line become disconnected. She assigned a staff nurse to special the patient, to closely monitor his vital signs, and draw blood gases as necessary. After discussing the need for close monitoring with the medical director, the charge nurse made arrangements for the patient to transfer to the intensive care area.	
The critical care nurse shall be cognizant of the radiation hazards present in the critical care environment and shall strive to minimize untoward effects on patients, visitors, and personnel.	The nursing staff in the respiratory care unit of Hospital A were concerned about the radiation hazard posed by the numerous portable chest x-rays being done. The head nurse consulted the Director of Diagnostic Radiology who conducted a three month study in the unit and concluded that there was negligible scatter from any of the portable x-ray units. He did advise, however, that a policy be drafted that any nurse who felt she was or could be pregnant be required to notify her head nurse so that appropriate precautions could be taken. However, in the coronary care unit, a great deal of fluoroscopy was being done for a research project and the Radiology Director felt it advisable to provide all nurses working in the CCU with the appropriate badges.	Joint Commission on Accreditation of Hospitals, *Accreditation Manual for Hospitals* 1980. Radiology Standard III Special Care Units Standard V Nursing Services Standard VI

COMPREHENSIVE STANDARD II: The critical care unit shall be constructed, equipped and operated in a manner which protects patients, visitors, and personnel from electrical hazards.

Supporting Standards	Examples of Implementation	References
The critical care unit construction, equipment, and operation shall comply with: —applicable building codes —state and/or federal occupational safety and health codes or standards —current Life Safety Codes of the National Fire Protection Association		Chisholm, L. A., R. Telden, and A. M. Dolan, Proceedings: A Patient Safety Program for Small Hospitals, *Biomedical Sciences Instrumentation*, 10:125–8, April, 1974. Dornette, W. H. Safety Standards and the Standard of Care, *Journal of Legal Medicine*. 2(6):49, Nov.–Dec., 1974.
A member of the critical care nursing staff shall participate in the selection of new equipment which will be used in the critical care area. Instruction by the vendor in use of new equipment shall be included as part of the purchase agreement.	The Critical Care Committee designated five of its members to participate in the purchasing of new cardiac monitoring equipment: two nurses, two physicians, and a biomedical engineer. Once the system was selected, all personnel were provided with initial instruction on its use and care. Upon installation, the vendor agreed to provide on-site instruction, around the clock, for seven days. Thereafter, equipment repair and consultative service was available on a 24 hour basis.	Feldtman, R. W., J. R. Derrick, Hospital Electrical Safety, *American Family Physician*, 13(3):127–37, March, 1976. Fischmann, G. S., S. R. Young, and E. S. Guttman, Engineering Medical Staff Department Heads Team up for Safety's Sake, *Hospitals*, 49(19):89, 92–3, October, 1975.

All electrical equipment and/or electronic systems used within the critical care unit shall be inspected for reliable and safe performance. Such inspection shall:
—be performed by a qualified person
—occur prior to initial use, after repair, and thereafter, at least semiannually
—be documented
	Several small hospitals in a rural community contracted with a biomedical engineering firm several miles away to provide:
	—periodic consultation regarding equipment purchases
	—inspection of new equipment prior to initial use
	—semiannual inspection of all electrical equipment and electronic systems
	—emergency consultation and equipment repair service
		Henning, Janet L., These are the Seven Danger Signals of Hospital Electrical Hazards, *Modern Hospital*, 121(1): 103–4, July, 1973.
		
		Joint Commission on the Accreditation of Hospitals, *Accreditation Manual*.
		  Standards for Special Care Units
		  Standards for Functional Safety and Sanitation
		
		Mylrea, K. C., and L. B. O'Neal, Electricity and Electrical Safety in the Hospital, *Nursing*, 6(1), 52–9, January 1976.

Supporting Standards	*Examples of Implementation*	*References*

Resource persons shall be available to the critical care staff at all times to provide advice and/or service on electrical equipment and electronic systems.

Information regarding the use and care of all equipment shall be readily available to the critical care staff.

Written policies and procedures regarding electrical safety shall be established. Such policies and procedures shall include, but not be limited to:

—preventive maintenance programs
—general precautions in the care of patients requiring the use of electrically operated devices
—precautions in the care of patients who are particularly prone to electrical hazards, such as those with:
  —debilitating conditions
  —loss of skin resistance
  —indwelling conductive catheters or cardiac leads
  —severe electrolyte imbalance
—proper grounding
—restrictions on the use of extension cords and adapters
—prevention of overload to any electrical system
—inspection of electrical equipment and electronic systems
—disposition and servicing of malfunctioning equipment
—regulation and maintenance of appropriate temperature and humidity to prevent electrical hazard

In the event of equipment failure, nurses in the above hospitals were to consult the written instructions accompanying the equipment kept on file at the nurses' station. If the problem was not solved, the biomedical engineering firm was to be notified for consultation and/or repair.

National Fire Protection Association Standards:
  NFPA 56A & 56B—Inhalation Anesthetics and Respiratory Therapy
  NFPA 70—National Electrical Code
  NFPA—Standard for Essential Electrical Systems for Health Care Facilities
  NFPA 76C—Recommended Practice on the Safe Use of High Frequency Electricity in Health Care Facilities

Parker, B., and S. A. Ritterman, An Inspection Procedure for Hospital Room Electrical Systems, *Medical Instrumentation* 9(2): 108–11, March–April, 1975.

Pfeiffer, E. A., A Simulator for Teaching Electrical Safety Procedures in the Hospital, *Medical Instrumentation*, 9(2): 103–5, March–April, 1975.

Sovie, M. D., and C. T. Fruehan, Protecting the Patient from Electrical Hazards. *Nursing Clinics of North America*, 7(3):469–480, September, 1972.

Standards for State and Local Health Department Applicable Codes and Regulations

Supporting Standards	Examples of Implementation	References
The critical care nurse shall demonstrate knowledge of and responsibility for implementation of an electrically safe environment and one which is consistent with established policy and procedure.	A number of critical care nurses noted excessive static electricity within the critical care unit. A humidity reading indicated a level of only 20% relative humidity. Since three patients in the unit were particularly prone to electrical hazard under such low humidity, an emergency call was made to the engineering department requesting repair of the unit's humidification system. Meanwhile, temporary methods of humidifying the environment were employed.	

COMPREHENSIVE STANDARD III: The critical care unit shall be constructed, equipped, and operated in a manner which protects patients, visitors, and personnel from fire hazard.

Supporting Standards	Examples of Implementation	References

The critical care unit construction, equipment, and operation shall comply with:
—applicable building codes
—fire prevention codes
—state and/or federal occupational safety and health codes or standards
—current Life Safety Codes of the National Fire Protection Association
		Joint Commission on the Accreditation of Hospitals *Accreditation Manual*.
		  Standards for Special Care Units
		  Standards for Functional Safety and Sanitation
		  Standards for Building Care Services

A manually operated fire alarm system shall be available within the critical care unit	At Hospital A, the critical care unit has a manually operated fire alarm centrally located in the nurses' station and one at the entrance of the unit. In the event of fire, patients are first removed from immediate danger; then the alarm is pulled, directly alerting the fire department. The person pulling the alarm or a designee is then responsible for notifying the hospital operator of the exact nature and location of the fire. The operator is in turn responsible for transmitting such information to the fire department, en route to the hospital.	National Fire Protection Association Standards: NFPA 3M—Hospital Emergency Preparedness NFPA 10—Installation, Maintenance, and Use of Portable Fire Extinguishers NFPA 56A—Inhalation Anesthetics
Fire extinguishers shall be available within the critical care unit at all times and shall be: —of the type required for the classes of fire anticipated in the critical care area —located so as to be readily available when needed —inspected at least monthly with the inspection documented	In a small community hospital, an A, B, and C rated fire extinguisher is located next to each fire alarm. At the first of each month, the head nurse is responsible for inspecting each extinguisher in the unit for proper pressure and pin placement. Inspection is documented on a small tag, directly attached to each extinguisher. In a large metropolitan hospital, a representative of the Hospital Safety Committee is responsible for such inspection and documentation.	NFPA 56B—Respiratory Therapy NFPA 70—National Electrical Code NFPA 56C—Standard for Laboratories in Health Related Institutions NFPA 56D—Standard for Hyperbaric Facilities NFPA 101—Life Safety Code NFPA 53M—Manual on Fire Hazards in Oxygen Enriched Atmospheres

Supporting Standards	*Examples of Implementation*	*References*

A member of the Critical Care Committee shall be a member of the Hospital Safety Committee.

A staff nurse from the critical care unit was appointed to represent the Critical Care Committee on the Hospital Safety Committee. To prepare, several references were acquired from the Biomedical Engineering Department in the hospital and from the State Health Department. In addition, the nursing administrator assisted in locating the appropriate JCAH standards.

The Critical Care Committee shall ensure that policies and procedures which will minimize fire hazards to patients, visitors, and personnel are established and reviewed annually. Such policies and procedures shall include, but not be limited to:
—prevention of fire hazards in the presence of an oxygen enriched atmosphere
—use, storage, and transportation of gas cylinders
—fire drills
—fire extinguishing system
—evacuation plan
—reporting of fire safety policy violations

The Safety Committee reviewed the NFPA caution related to the potential fire hazard involved in defibrillation during oxygen administration. The committee recommended appropriate alteration of the cardiac resuscitation procedure so as to prevent the fire hazard. The staff nurse informed the Critical Care Committee of the recommendation, and the procedure was altered accordingly. Plans were made to inform all critical care personnel of the potential hazard and the policy change.

Dornette, W. H., Safety Standards and the Standard of Care, *Journal of Legal Medicine*, 2(6); 49, November–December, 1974.

Farman, J. V., Fire Risks in Intensive Care Units and Operating Theaters: Evacuation of Surgical Patients, *Proceedings of the Royal Society of Medicine*, 69(8), 603–4, August, 1976.

Perrin, J. Is Your Hospital Ready for a Fire? *Dimensions of Health Services*, 53(5), 14–5, 17, May, 1976.

Fire drills shall be held at least quarterly for each shift, their occurrence documented and evaluated, and corrective action taken for any deficiency.

After each quarterly fire drill, the nurse in charge submits a brief report including deficiencies and corrective action taken. Each report is kept on file, and a copy forwarded to the Critical Care Committee.

The critical care nurse shall demonstrate knowledge of and responsibility for implementation of all aspects of the fire safety program.

As part of each fire drill, nurses are asked to demonstrate their knowledge of randomly selected policies and procedures related to fire safety. For example, nurses may be asked to:
—locate the oxygen cut-off valve

Supporting Standards	Examples of Implementation	References
	—describe the proper use of a fire extinguisher —relate the steps in the fire evacuation plan In addition, each nurse is evaluated on his/her ability to implement the fire safety program, as part of the formal periodic performance appraisal.	

COMPREHENSIVE STANDARD IV: The critical care unit shall have essential equipment and supplies immediately available at all times.

Supporting Standards	Examples of Implementation	References
The critical care nurse shall participate in establishing an inventory of necessary equipment and supplies for each unit that will: —include routine as well as emergency equipment —reflect the specific needs of the potential patient population —be reviewed annually	Inventories of supplies will vary depending on the patient population of the unit and the average daily census. Although the inventory levels are reviewed yearly, the staff should discuss them periodically to ensure adequacy at all times	Adler, D., and N. Shoemaker, (eds.) *Organization and Management of Critical Care Facilities.* St. Louis: C. V. Mosby Co., 1979. Burrell, Jeb L., and L. Burrell, *Intensive Nursing Care.* St. Louis: C. V. Mosby Co., 1969. Bushnell, S. S., *Respiratory Intensive Care Nursing.* Boston: Little, Brown and Co., 1973. Huether, Sue, Biomedical Instrumentation and the Nurse Practitioner, *Nursing Clinics of North America*, 13(4), December, 1978. Joint Commission on Accreditation of Hospitals, *Accreditation Manual*, Standards for Special Care Units.
The critical care nurse shall participate in establishing written policies and procedures for ordering, monitoring, and replacing equipment and supplies needed for each unit.	In a large medical center, a system for monitoring inventory levels and automatic restocking might be the responsibility of the appropriate ancillary department, e.g., Central Supply, Pharmacy, Housekeeping, and Dietary. However, in a smaller community hospital, it might be a nursing service responsibility to monitor inventory levels and to notify the appropriate department when additional or nonroutine supplies are needed.	
The critical care nurse shall ensure that equipment and supplies considered necessary during emergency situations shall: —be centrally located and readily accessible, and —have documented inspection at least daily by appropriate personnel	Whether restocking emergency drugs and equipment is done by the nursing service or another department, it is the critical care nurse's responsibility to ensure that these roles and accountabilities are clearly defined so that appropriate equipment and drugs are available in an emergency situation.	Kinney, J. M., et al, *Manual of Surgical Intensive Care.* Philadelphia: W. B. Saunders Co., 1977, Chapters 3, 5, and 6. Skillman, J. J., ed., *Intensive Care.* Boston: Little, Brown and Co., 1975.
The critical care nurse shall be responsible for ensuring the availability of necessary supplies and equipment before admission of a new patient.	While receiving a telephone report on a patient with chest trauma being admitted through the emergency room, the critical care nurse determined that appropriate equipment to care for this patient was not present in the unit. The critical care nurse	

Supporting Standards	*Examples of Implementation*	*References*
	could not assume responsibility for this patient until the appropriate equipment was available. Therefore, the nurse asked the emergency room to delay transferring the patient until the necessary ventilator, chest suction pumps, and infusion controllers could be obtained.	
Provision shall be made for replenishment of needed supplies on a 24 hour basis.	In some hospitals, supply areas may be staffed on a 24 hour basis. In many other hospitals, replenishing supplies may be either the responsibility of an on-call person who can be reached by the hospital operator, or the responsibility of the nursing supervisor on duty.	
The critical care nurse shall demonstrate knowledge of and responsibility for obtaining necessary equipment and supplies.		

COMPREHENSIVE STANDARD V: The critical care unit shall have a comprehensive infection control program.

Supporting Standards	Examples of Inplementation	References
Written infection control policies and procedures specific to the unit shall be established and shall comply with any requirements directed by: —national, state, and local agencies —hospital infection control committee —physical layout of the unit Written infection control policies and procedures shall address the prevention and control of infection among patients, personnel, and visitors. These shall include, but not be limited to: —patient eligibility for admission, including requirements for equipment and personnel —methods employed in the prevention of potential nosocomial infections	Some procedures are commonly associated with nosocomial infections. Therefore, policies should be developed for definitive techniques involved in preventing infections related to such procedures (including but not limited to) as: —intravenous therapy —urinary catheters —tracheal suctioning —respiratory therapy equipment —dialysis equipment	Allen, J. C., ed., *Infection and the Compromised Host*. Baltimore: Williams & Wilkens, 1976. Bennett, J. V., and Brachman, P. S., *Hospital Infections*. Boston: Little, Brown & Co., 1979. Burke, J. F., and G. Y. Hildick, *The Infection Prone Patient*. Boston: Little, Brown & Co., 1978. Dubay, E. and R. Grubb, *Infection Prevention and Control*. St. Louis: C. V. Mosby, 1978. *Isolation Techniques for Use in Hospitals*, U.S. Department of Health, Education, and Welfare, Center for Disease Control, 1975. Meshelany, C., *Infection Control Manual*. Oradell, N.J.: Medical Economics Co., Book Division, 1976. Official Report of the American Public Health Association (12th Ed.), Beneson, A. S., ed., *Control of Communicable Diseases in Man*, 1975. Ramsay, A. M., *Infectious Diseases*. London: Heinemann, 1978.
—storage, handling, and disposal of supplies, waste, and equipment —control of traffic (hospital personnel and visitors) in the critical care unit and isolation areas —inspection for outdated sterile items —environmental disinfection and equipment sterilization —nursing personnel assignment —apparel worn by hospital personnel	Common items that require procedures regarding their storage, handling, and disposal are gloves, dressings, tissues, urine, feces, linen, equipment, instruments, and disposable items	

Supporting Standards	*Examples of Implementation*	*References*
—specific indications for isolation/precaution requirements in relation to potential or actual diagnosis	Specific indications for isolation/precaution requirements would include: type of room; necessity and storage of gown, gloves, masks, sphygmomanometer, stethoscope, needles, syringes, dressings, tissues, thermometers, linen, and dishes; storage of patient's clothing and personal effects; disposition of laboratory specimens, linen, equipment, instruments, dressings, urine, and feces as well as other waste; transportation of patients, visitors; concurrent and terminal cleaning for each of the following categories: —strict isolation —respiratory isolation —protective isolation —enteric isolation —wound and skin precautions —blood precautions —excretion precautions —secretion precautions	
—responsibility and authority for initiating and enforcing infection control	At 3:00 p.m., a 21-month-old child was admitted to Hospital D's five bed pediatric intensive care unit for status asthmaticus requiring mechanical ventilation. Later on that evening, the baby's temperature began to rise and maculopapular lesions appeared on his chest, abdomen, and back. On questioning, the mother stated that her other child had just "gotten over chicken pox." When notified, the physician stated he would be in later that evening to review the case. The nurse, concerned about the possibility of infecting the other children in the unit, notified the supervisor and the infection control practitioner.	

Supporting Standards	Examples of Implementation	References
	A decision was made to transfer the baby to strict isolation in a private room on the general pediatric floor and staffing was rearranged to provide critical care nurses to care for the baby in this room. The physician was notified of this decision.	
—acceptable ventilation patterns, air exchange rates, air temperature, and humidity		
The Critical Care Committee, in collaboration with the Hospital Infection Control Committee, shall annually review and revise the unit's infection control policies and procedures.		
The Critical Care Committee and the Hospital Infection Control Committee shall devise an ongoing system for reporting, reviewing, and evaluating infections within the critical care unit.	The Critical Care Committee might include a member of the Infection Control Committee. Time should be allotted on each agenda for discussion of infection control issues, discussion of serious problems, sharing of new concepts/techniques, and planning for prevention of potential problems as they relate to the critical care unit.	
The Critical Care Committee shall monitor all findings from concurrent and retrospective patient care evaluations that relate to infection control activities within the critical care unit.	The hospital Patient Care Evaluation Committee conducted an audit on urinary tract infections. The committee found a high incidence of urinary tract infections among patients with indwelling urinary catheters who had been cared for in the medical intensive care unit.	
	This information was referred to the Critical Care Committee for investigation. They found that careful handwashing was not consistently performed by the staff providing direct patient care in the unit.	

Supporting Standards	Examples of Implementation	References
	Appropriate corrective action was taken and the findings and action reported to the hospital Patient Care Evaluation Committee.	
The quality of patient care shall be maintained regardless of the patient's need for isolation.	Mr. C was brought to the emergency room of Hospital Y with full thickness burns of his neck, right arm and hand, and partial thickness burns of his chest. He was in acute respiratory distress requiring mechanical ventilation.	
	Hospital Y is not equipped to handle severely burned patients because the structure of its intensive care unit precludes reverse isolation within the unit. Therefore, patients like Mr. C are transferred to Hospital X's burn unit; however, Hospital X had no available beds. A private room on a general unit was prepared and equipped to care for Mr. C with a critical care nurse assigned to each shift. A nurse from the general unit was assigned each shift to assist the critical care nurse.	
The critical care unit orientation shall include: —introduction to the institution's infection control program —individual responsibilities for prevention and control of infection	The critical care orientation program in Hospital A included a presentation on infection control by the infection control practitioner. The presentation included: —the role of the critical care nurse in the prevention, reporting, and control of infection —hospital and unit infection control policies and procedures —formal and informal lines of communication relative to responsibilities and authority for intervention —necessary documentation concerning potential or actual infections —current pharmacologic interventions	

Supporting Standards	Examples of Implementation	References
Documented inservice education concerning current infection control practices, pharmacologic interventions, and their nursing implications shall be provided.	In Hospital B all nursing personnel are required to view the videotapes on infection control. However, Hospital C has limited resources. Therefore, the head nurse of the critical care unit selected and made available several current articles on the prevention and control of infectious diseases.	
The critical care nurse shall demonstrate —knowledge of the classifications of infectious conditions requiring isolation or precaution —responsibility for implementation of infection control policies and procedures	While changing a post-op abdominal dressing the ICU nurse noted the patient's wound was reddened, warm, and draining a "milky" liquid. The old dressings had a foul odor. The nurse obtained a wound culture per standing order, placed the patient on wound and skin precautions, and notified the attending physician.	
Infection control resources shall be readily available.	Infection control resources could include: —professional staff such as a microbiologist or nurse epidemiologist —infectious disease textbook —pharmacology textbook —Center for Disease Control publications —relevant policy and procedures manuals	

COMPREHENSIVE STANDARD VI: The critical care unit shall be managed in a manner which ensures the delivery of safe and effective care to the critically ill.

Supporting Standards	Examples of Implementation	References
The critical care unit shall have a written philosophy and objectives which —reflect the nursing service philosophy and objectives, and —guide the nursing activities of the unit. The operations of the unit shall conform to local, state, and federal laws. The activities of the critical care unit shall be under the direction of a multidisciplinary committee, with appropriate representation from the medical and nursing staffs and other support services directly involved with the critically ill patient.	Shortly after being hired to work in a large medical-surgical intensive care unit R. G. asked to attend the next meeting of the Critical Care Committee to more quickly acquire a working knowledge of the unit operations. The head nurse informed R. G. of the time and date of the next meeting and provided an agenda of topics to be discussed. R. G. attended the meeting and noted representation from respiratory therapy, pharmacy, dietary, social work, and physical therapy, as well as the medical and nursing co-directors.	Adler, D., and Shoemaker, N. eds., *AACN Organization and Management of Critical Care Facilities*. St. Louis: C. V. Mosby Co., 1979, Chapters 2, 3, 7, 8, 9, 11. Joint Commission on Accreditation of Hospitals, *Accreditation Manual*, Standards for Special Care Units.
A policy and procedures manual shall be developed, annually reviewed, and approved by the Critical Care Committee, subject to approval by the hospital administration. Where appropriate, other non-nursing departments shall participate in the development of these policies and procedures. These shall include, but not be limited to: —patient admission and discharge criteria —use of standing orders —decision-making roles of staff		

Supporting Standards	Examples of Implementation	References
—evaluation methods to determine effectiveness of the unit —ongoing requirements for continuing education of professional staff —regulation of visitors —regulations for traffic control —safety practices for patients, staff, and visitors —role of the unit in hospital disaster plans —procedures for maintenance and repair of equipment —patient care procedures, including specification of personnel to perform these procedures —housekeeping procedures —infection control measures —list of necessary equipment for the unit —electrical safety regulations —fire safety regulations —medication administration —patient consultation and referral mechanisms —discharge planning —patient and family teaching —documentation of the nursing care given —maintenance of required records, reports, or statistical information —scope of activity of volunteers or paid attendants —initiation and termination of life-sustaining measures		
The critical care unit budget shall be developed and administered by the medical and nursing directors.	The head nurse and medical director of the intensive care unit at this hospital meet monthly to review the budget. They identified a need for replacing an ECG machine and developed a proposal which was submitted to administration for approval.	

COMPREHENSIVE STANDARD VII: The critical care unit shall have appropriately qualified staff to provide care on a twenty-four hour basis.

Supporting Standards	Examples of Implementation	References
Professional nursing staff shall possess the following qualifications: —current license —documentation of the acquisition of a knowledge base with attendant psychomotor skills common to and requisite for the care of the critically ill —willingness to participate in continuing education as indicated by past record —current individual malpractice insurance		
Potential staff shall be interviewed by the critical care nurse manager for appropriateness of employment.	While reviewing the policy on personnel staffing, R. G. reflected on the application for a position in that unit. Although the unit had been short-staffed, R. G. had been interviewed by both the head nurse and supervisor of the unit, and was asked many questions regarding: —patient populations R. G. had previously cared for in other critical care units —previous participation in continuing education activities —past involvement and willingness to engage in learning/teaching activities with peers or patients —personal use of the nursing process in selected patient care situations —personal, professional, and ethical values R. G.'s general impression of the hiring process indicated there was concern for the nurse's level of expertise and for maintaining quality patient care, even though staffing was low.	

Supporting Standards	*Examples of Implementation*	*References*
All professional nursing staff shall demonstrate knowledge of and responsibility for the implementation of the unit's policies and procedures.		
There shall be sufficient professional nursing personnel to provide effective patient care. The nurse–patient ratio shall reflect recognition of the patient's acuity and required nursing care. Staffing patterns shall be reviewed regularly by the Critical Care Committee to ensure the delivery of safe care.	The recent shortage of professional nursing staff, coupled with a marked increase in patient acuity levels, created much concern about the quality of patient care in R. G.'s unit. Because unit policy required that only nurses who had completed the unit's orientation program could independently deliver care in the unit, the Critical Care Committee recommended closure of two beds. Hospital administration concurred with the recommendation and closed the beds for a 2-month period at which time the situation was to be reexamined	
Unit staff shall participate in the development of staffing patterns. These patterns shall provide for: —the flexibility to provide optimum patient care on a 24-hour basis —utilization of at least 50% RN staff on each shift —restriction of unlicensed personnel from direct delivery of nursing care (except nursing students, with an instructor present at all times) —provisions for unit staff to function intermittently in a support role in other areas, but guaranteeing prompt return to their primary unit when needed —contingency plans to ensure availability of qualified critical care nursing staff		

COMPREHENSIVE STANDARD VIII: The critical care nurse shall be competent and current in critical care nursing.

Supporting Standards	Examples of Implementation	References
Prior to assuming independent responsibility for patient care the critical care nurse shall demonstrate possession of the knowledge base requisite for the care of the critically ill. This knowledge base shall include that content necessary for: —collection and processing of data related to the physiological and psychosocial status of the critically ill person —identification and determination of the priority of the patient's problems/needs —development of a plan of nursing care —implementation of the plan of nursing care —evaluation of care delivered	During a designated orientation a critical care orientee could demonstrate possession of the requisite knowledge base through successful completion of any of the following: —a formal critical care nursing course —critical care nursing challenge examinations —certification in critical care nursing —critical care programmed study course —oral exam developed by the health care institution	AACN's Clinical Reference for Critical Care Nursing. (To be published in 1980). AACN's Core Curriculum for Critical Care Nursing, 1975; revised edition. AACN's Methods in Critical Care. (To be published in 1980). American Heart Association, CPR Guidelines. American Nurses' Association Standards of Nursing Practice. Cardiovascular Council, American Heart Association, Standards of Cardiovascular Nursing. Lancour, Jane, Legal Aspects of Critical Care Nursing, Nursing Clinics of North America, 9(3), Philadelphia: W. B. Saunders, 435–444, September, 1974.
Prior to assuming independent responsibility for patient care, the critical care nurse shall demonstrate possession of psychomotor skills common to and requisite for care of the critically ill.	During a designated orientation program, a critical care orientee might complete a skills list by the following methods: —manipulation of patient care equipment and performance of assessment techniques in a simulated setting and/or —manipulation of patient care equipment and performance of assessment techniques under direct supervision in a clinical area	Mann, James K., Nursing Leadership in the Critical Care Setting. Nursing Clinics of North America, 13(1). Philadelphia: W. B. Saunders Co., March, 1978, 137, 131–138
Prior to assuming independent responsibility for patient care, the critical care nurse shall demonstrate in supervised clinical practice the ability to integrate knowledge and psychomotor skills through applications of the nursing process and subsequent documentation.	A 70-bed rural hospital, with three critical care beds, has developed an orientation program for ICU-CCU nurses. Each orientee completes a list of behavioral objectives while working with an experienced nurse in the unit. The orientee makes daily patient rounds with the nurse-	

Supporting Standards	*Examples of Implementation*	*References*

preceptor and physicians during which time he/she learns some patient assessment techniques, pathophysiology with associated signs and symptoms, medical therapy, and nursing care. The orientee has supervised practice in certain procedures for one hour 3 times weekly and is expected to complete programmed instruction in dysrhythmias, CCU nursing, fluid and electrolytes, drugs, and decision-making situations. At the completion of orientation, the orientee presents a patient care plan to the unit nursing staff to demonstrate the decision-making process, correlation of theory and practice, and concern for the emotional needs of the patient and family. The orientee receives an end-of-orientation evaluation from the nurse-preceptor and head nurse; at this time, areas which need further study are identified. The length of orientation is flexible, based on the needs of the nurse.

Critical care nurses shall be responsible for seeking educational resources and creating learning experiences necessary for achievement and maintenance of currency in their areas of practice. Such experiences may include, but are not limited to, the following:

—independent study
—nursing preceptorship
—inservice classes and grand rounds
—formal orientation
—academic classes
—seminars and symposiums
—rotating assignments under supervision

J. H., who has worked in the ICU-CCU of S.L. Hospital for 6 months, recognized a need for additional learning experiences to improve his critical care knowledge and skills. Since the current inservice classes were not meeting his individual needs, he elected to develop his own plan. After reviewing the ICU-CCU patient population, his patient care experiences, and his strengths and weaknesses, J. H. developed goals and a study plan. The plan included a three hour physiology course, one seminar on crisis intervention in the critical

Supporting Standards	Examples of Implementation	References
—affiliation with another institution for a specific learning objective —tutoring by a nurse consultant —patient rounds with members of other disciplines	care setting, and journal reading. At the completion of three months, J. H. evaluated his progress toward his preset goals.	
Additional knowledge and skills shall be acquired prior to assuming a responsibility for the care of patient populations for which the nurse has not been prepared. Characteristics of patient population to consider: —disease modality —treatment modality —age of patients —acuity	If an area designated for medical cardiology is expanded to include surgical cardiology, the nurses' scope of knowledge and skills will need to expand accordingly. Should the unit be further expanded to include pediatric as well as adult patients, a still greater depth of knowledge would be required to provide safe care.	

COMPREHENSIVE STANDARD IX: The critical care nurse's performance appraisal shall be based upon the roles and responsibilities identified in the job description.

Supporting Standards	Examples of Implementation	References
Job descriptions shall be criterion-based, written and readily available for each classification of nursing personnel, and shall include: —job title —organizational relationships —basic functions and responsibilities —requirements and special skills needed —expectations for continuing education		
Nursing staff shall be evaluated at the end of the orientation period, at the end of the probationary period, and at least yearly thereafter, or as needed.	At the end of orientation, R. G. met with the head nurse and clinical specialist to review progress in meeting orientation objectives. Although the hospital probationary period was completed, R. G. understood the ICU probationary period was 6 months and that reevaluation would occur at 3 and at 6 months to determine permanent employment in the ICU. During this evaluation, the three individuals reviewed progress to date and established continuing objectives for the remainder of the probationary period. The three agreed that R. G. was doing well but required additional skills in dysrhythmia interpretation. It was decided that R. G. would attend a workshop on dysrhythmias in the near future.	
Nursing staff shall be evaluated by a variety of mechanisms. These mechanisms may include evaluation by: —self	The following are examples of methods by which proficiency may be evaluated. —self-evaluation might be performed on a daily basis by the critical care nurse. This evaluation could be accomplished by: —initiating group discus-	

Supporting Standards	Examples of Implementation	References
	—researching pertinent literature —case presentations —utilizing audit criteria —utilizing AACN's *Standards for Care of Critically Ill*	
—supervisor	—evaluation could be performed regularly by a qualified supervisor. This evaluation could be informal or formal and might include: —objective review of verbal patient care reports —nursing rounds —discussion of orders for medications, diets, or therapies —formal overall nursing evaluations, written by a qualified supervisor —mutual evaluations performed by the critical care nurse and a qualified supervisor —revew of skills list with documentation of improved skills and areas that require practice.	
—peers	—evaluation could be performed on a monthly basis for the entire critical care nusing staff through: —verification from peers or clinicians from other disciplines —staff meetings —support group sessions with psychiatrist/psychologist or psychiatric clinical specialist during which staff and patient needs and problems are discussed —morbidity and mortality conferences —case presentations —review of quality assurance data —scheduled inservice classes —simulated clinical situations —gathering data or statistics	

COMPREHENSIVE STANDARD X: The critical care unit shall have a well-defined, organized, written program to evaluate care of the critically ill.

Supporting Standards	Examples of Implementation	References
The evaluation program shall reflect the following: —current scientific knowledge —professional and personal values	The entire document, *Standards for Nursing Care of the Critically Ill*, has as its purpose evaluation of care. As such, implementation of the Evaluation Standard is well demonstrated in various sections throughout this document.	American Nurses' Association. *A Plan for Implementation of the Standards of Nursing Practice*. Kansas City, Mo.: The American Nurses' Association, 1975.
The evaluation program shall include identified standards for care and criteria for achieving the stated standards.	The standards and criteria are specifically identified in Part II-A, Structure Standards and Part II-B, Process Standards. It is also possible to evaluate using outcome standards/criteria, and although these are not specifically stated in this document, methods of developing outcomes are addressed in Part II-C, Outcome Standards.	American Nurses' Association. *Guidelines for Review of Nursing Care at the Local Level*. Kansas City, Mo.: The American Nurses' Association, 1976. American Nurses' Association. *Quality Assurance Workbook*. Kansas City, Mo.: The American Nurses' Association, 1976. Lang, N. M., Are Professional Nurses Ready for a Quality Assurance Program?, *Nursing Outlook*, November, 1970, 18:24–32.
Measurements needed to determine the degree of standard and criteria attainment shall be obtained. Strengths and weaknesses shall be identified through interpretation of the measurements.	Part III, Implementation of Standards, addresses the many methods that may be used to determine attainment of standards and criteria. Strengths and weaknesses are identified as a result of these methods, and appropriate courses of action are selected and implemented.	
Possible courses of action based on the findings shall be identified and course(s) of action taken. Action(s) shall be taken. Reevaluation shall occur.	It is perhaps most appropriate to view the evaluation criteria as illustrated in the circular diagram in Part I, The Evolution and Philosophy of the Standards. Evaluation is viewed here as an ongoing, continuous process.	

COMPREHENSIVE STANDARD XI: Critical care nursing practice shall include both the conduct and utilization of clinical research.

Supporting Standards	Examples of Implementation	References
The critical care nurse shall conduct and utilize research independently and/or in collaboration with others. Such activities should reflect: —support and encouragement of nursing colleagues who are engaged in clinical research —an awareness of one's strengths and limitations in various aspects of the research process —current knowledge of clinical research in one's field of practice —respect for a variety of types of research efforts, each of which can further the development of nursing knowledge	A staff nurse in the critical care unit began to notice respiratory distress in several patients during endotracheal suctioning. These observations were shared with the head nurse, who supported the nurse and encouraged further investigation. Both nurses decided to examine their observations more closely and to gather additional information about suctioning procedures, including procedure manuals, nursing and medical literature, research reports and consultants. It was determined that a great deal of controversy existed concerning proper suctioning techniques and the rationale behind each. However, one particular study demonstrated that a specific suctioning procedure was superior to other methods in reducing respiratory distress and increasing oxygenation during suctioning. Recognizing their lack of research skills, the two nurses contacted a nurse researcher and a clinical nurse specialist with expertise in respiratory nursing to assist them in examining the specific study and to determine subsequent steps necessary to solve the problem they had identified. Together, they concluded that while the initial study demonstrated positive results, further investigation was needed to validate the results and to assure that the suctioning procedure was safe for use.	Aydelotte, M. K., Nursing Research in Clinical Settings: Problems and Issues, *Sigma Theta Tau Reflections*. March, 1976, Vol. 2, 3–6. Batey, M. V., Research: Its Dissemination and Utilization in Nursing·Practice, *Washington State Journal of Nursing*, Winter, 1976, 6–9. Diers, D., This I believe about nursing research, *Nursing Outlook*, Nov. 1970, 18, 50–54. Lysaught, J. P., *An Abstract for Action*. New York: McGraw-Hill, 1970, 83–87. Notter, L. E. The Vital Significance of Clinical Nursing Research, *Cardiovascular Nursing*. September–October, 1972, 8(5), 19–22.

Supporting Standards	*Examples of Implementation*	*References*
	Several members of the critical care nursing staff became interested in the study to validate the effects of the suctioning procedure and worked collaboratively with the nurse researcher and nurse specialist to: —identify the exact problem for study —identify the design of the study, including specification of the suctioning procedure and methods of measuring its effects —select or construct tools to be used for measurement or for data collection —identify means of gaining patient consent to participate in the study —seek approval from the hospital Research Ethics Committee	Brink, P. J., and Wood, M. J., *Basic Steps in Planning Nursing Research*. North Scituate, Mass: Duxbury Press, 1978.
The critical care nurse shall facilitate current and future clinical research through the consistent and accurate recording of data related to the patient's condition and nursing care provided. Such data should include, but not be limited to: —physiological status —psychosocial status	Once the study was ready for implementation, all nurses participated in the collection of data, each recognizing the necessity of complete accuracy and strict adherence to the study design. Blood gases were drawn at specific time intervals before and after suctioning; cardiac monitoring was performed for specified time periods just prior to, during, and after suctioning; observations of patient color, distress, and anxiety levels were made at specific intervals, using predefined rating scales.	
The critical care nurse shall implement changes in clinical practice only when the safety and effectiveness of the new practice have been established through an adequate research base and systematic investigation. Such changes must be accompanied by:	The data, when analyzed and reviewed, demonstrated findings similar to those of the initial study. This validated the initial findings, and it was concluded that the suctioning procedure was indeed effective and safe for use. The nurses then took the neces-	

Supporting Standards	Examples of Implementation	References
—a written policy change —incorporation into an on-going evaluation system or mechanism	sary steps to incorporate the new suctioning procedure into the hospital's official policies and procedures.	
The critical care nurse shall explore methods of sharing the findings of research efforts with nursing colleagues and with those from other disciplines.	Finally, the nurses identified two methods of sharing their findings with other colleagues. These included a publication and a presentation of the study report at a regional nursing conference.	
The critical care nurse shall determine the potential hazards and benefits related to research involving subjects for whom she/he is responsible, including —patients —family or significant others —personnel	At a routine staff meeting, a memorandum was read to inform the unit nurses of a research study which was to be implemented the following month. The study involved a "new and exciting combination of intravenous solutions to be used for patients in cardiac failure." A physiologist from a nearby university was the principal investigator and two cardiologists from the hospital staff were also involved. The nurses requested additional information, including reference materials, a summary of potential hazards and possible benefits, and any developed protocols or consent forms.	American Nurses' Association. *Code for Nurses with Interpretative Statements.* Kansas City, Mo.: The American Nurses' Association, 1976. American Nurses' Association. *Human Rights Guidelines for Nurses in Clinical and Other Research.* Kansas City, Mo.: The American Nurses' Association, 1975. American Nurses' Association, Research and Studies Committee, The Nurse in Research; ANA Guidelines on Ethical Values. *Nursing Research*, March–April, 1968, 17, 104–107.
The critical care nurse shall act to protect the rights of human subjects, including: —the right to privacy and confidentiality —the right to voluntary and informed consent without coercion —the right to freedom from mental and emotional harm —the right to know any potential harm or benefits related to participation in the research —the right to refuse to participate or to withdraw from a study without fearing reprisal or jeopardizing care	After reviewing the requested materials, staff invited the researchers to discuss several areas of concern. At the meeting, the researchers stated that there was no need to obtain patient consent. The nurses left the meeting with serious concerns about patient safety and violation of subjects' human rights.	Arminger, S. B., Ethics of Nursing Research, *Nursing Research*, September–October, 1977, 26, 330–336. Carper, B. A., The Ethics of Caring, *Advances in Nursing Science*, April 1979, 1, 11–19. Creighton, H., Legal Concerns of Nursing Research, *Nursing Research*, Sept–Oct, 1977, 26, 337–341. Curtin, L. L., The Nurse as Advocate: A Philosophical Foundation for Nursing, *Advances in Nursing Science*, April 1979, 1, 1–10. Sigman, P., Ethical Choice in Nursing, *Advances in Nursing Science*, April 1979, 1, 37–52.

Supporting Standards	*Examples of Implementation*	*References*
The critical care nurse shall be cognizant of and may participate in the mechanisms available to address violation of the rights of human subjects.	The head nurse explained the staff's concerns to the director of nursing, and together they met with the chairperson at the nearby university. They were told by the chairperson that a review was indeed necessary before the investigators could initiate their study. They were assured that the ethical review would be conducted immediately and that they would receive notification of the results. The director and head nurse were encouraged to develop a mechanism within their own agency so that resolution of similar problems could be handled more easily and could reflect the agency's own philosophy and goals. The director of nursing initiated efforts to develop a method of addressing similar problems. Meanwhile, the head nurse worked with the staff to determine their responsibility in the protection of critically ill patients from violation of their human rights. The state nurses' association served as a resource to the staff and provided a variety of educational materials which were incorporated into the unit's orientation program for new nurses.	

Supporting Standards	Examples of Implementation	References
	It is imperative that the critical care nurse be aware of those instances where either nursing or medical actions may result in a lawsuit.	Creighton, H., *Law Every Nurse Should Know*. Philadelphia: W. B. Saunders, 1977. Sarner, Harvey, *The Nurse and the Law*. Philadelphia: W. B. Saunders, 1969. Willig, Sidney, *The Nurse's Guide to the Law*. New York: McGraw-Hill Book Co., 1970.
Patients shall be fully advised in advance of all nursing and/or medical procedures to which they are subjected, signing a written informed consent when required. Related causes of action: Assault: An intentional act which places victim in apprehension of injury.	A suit for assault could result from the manner with which a critical care nurse approaches a belligerent and hostile patient demanding a prn narcotic. If the nurse approaches the patient holding the syringe in a threatening gesture, the patient could perceive it as an intent to harm.	
Battery: An intentionally harmful or offensive touching without consent of victim.	Battery suits have resulted when a surgeon has performed a nonemergent laparotomy on a patient without first obtaining an informed consent.	
Patients shall be allowed freedom of movement within their hospital room and are allowed to discharge themselves from the hospital. Related causes of action: False Imprisonment: An intentional act which results in victim's confinement within boundaries set by wrongful party.	This may occur when a nurse refuses to allow a critically ill patient to leave the hospital even though the patient has signed the "against medical advice" form. Another instance would be when a patient is placed in leather restraints by a nurse without a physician's order and without notifying the physician.	

Supporting Standards	*Examples of Implementation*	*References*

Patients shall receive nursing care in accordance with good nursing practice and those policies specifically established by the hospital.

Related causes of action:

Negligence: A breach of a duty of due care which proximately causes injury to victim. Malpractice is the negligence of a professional. Required elements of negligence:

—duty of care (e.g., to perform nursing functions according to nursing policy manual);

—departure from duty (nurse fails to act in accordance with policy);

—damages resulted to the patient (patient suffers from monetary loss);

—causal connection between the departure and injury can be demonstrated (patient injured because nurse failed to adhere to nursing policy).

Negligence occurs when a nurse, in violation of a nursing policy, does not check a medication card against the physician's order sheet, and thereby gives a wrong medication to the patient. If this results in damage to the patient, e.g. a longer hospital stay, an adverse reaction, etc., then the wrong action has met all four elements for negligence.

Another example would be if a nurse failed to check a unit of blood with another nurse or physician, as required by nursing policy, and the patient was transfused with unmatched blood.

Patients shall be assured that any medical information will be shared only with health professionals treating the patient and that any other communication is restricted or occurs only with the consent of the patient.

Related causes of action:

Defamation: Invasion of victim's interest in reputation and good name by wrongful party intentionally communicating matter to third party (libel is defamation reduced to written or printed form; slander is oral defamation).

Defamation may occur when a nurse discloses information about patients; for example, if the nurse discusses a patient's psychiatric evaluation with the patient's roommate.

Suit might also result if the nurse communicated to newspaper reporters that the famous parents of a pediatric patient were actually known child abusers.

COMPREHENSIVE STANDARD XII: *(Continued)*

Supporting Standards	*Examples of Implementation*	*References*
The patient's family members shall not be subjected to: —incorrect information concerning the patient —careless treatment of the patient Related cause of action: Infliction of Mental Distress: Intentional act results in subjecting victim to an emotional shock which is demonstrated by physical injury	A critical care nurse was sued when the nurse informed a pregnant wife that her husband, who had only been slightly injured in an automobile accident, was "not expected to live." This news resulted in the wife's miscarriage. A lawsuit could result from the actions of a nurse who, in the presence of the mother, carelessly lost her grip on a newborn infant. Even if the infant was not injured, the action could result in a mental shock to the mother and the nurse could be subject to suit.	
Patients shall be treated in a dignified manner; only those professionals directly involved in their care have access to their medical information; and this information will not be released or disclosed to others without their approval. Related cause of action: Invasion of Privacy: Using a victim's name or likeness for commercial use, intruding into the victim's private life, or disclosing private facts about the victim to the public.	Allowing an unidentified and/or unauthorized person to read the medical chart of a patient could result in an invasion of privacy suit against the nurse. A suit could also result if a nurse disclosed to a friend next door that a neighborhood girl just had an abortion performed at the hospital.	

PROCESS
STANDARDS

Part II-B

VALUE STATEMENT: The critical care nurse shall utilize the nursing process in the delivery of patient care.

COMPREHENSIVE STANDARD I: Data shall be collected continuously on all critically ill patients wherever they may be located.

Supporting Standards	Examples of Implementation	
	Respiratory	*Cardiovascular*
	A 62 year old caucasian female is admitted with a provisional diagnosis of acute respiratory failure; rule out pneumonia.	A 49 year old male is admitted with a provisional diagnosis of severe congestive heart failure.
The critical care nurse shall collect subjective and objective data to determine the gravity of the patient's problems/needs.	ECG monitoring was initiated and the rhythm strip showed sinus tachycardia with 1–2 multifocal premature ventricular beats per min. BP 150/90 mmHg right arm; 142/86 mmHg left arm. Apical heart rate 130/min, irregular. Grunting respirations, 40/min, irregular and gasping, with use of accessory muscles. Breathing through pursed lips with intermittent weak nonproductive cough; oxygen per face mask at 40% $F_I O_2$. Head of bed in full upright position. Diffuse wheezes throughout both lung fields; crackles heard bilaterally at level of scapulae and below. Patient stated in gasping breaths, "I can't catch my breath; please help me!"	*General appearance:* patient easily arousable and oriented to time, person, and place. Skin color very pale and nailbeds cyanotic. Head of bed elevated 60°. *Cardiac status:* BP 110/70 mm Hg. Heart rate 90/min. Cardiac monitoring was initiated using Modified Chest Lead I–sinus rhythm with premature ventricular contractions occurring 10/min. Neck veins distended 8 cm above the angle of Louis. S_3 gallop at apex. Bilateral ankle edema. Dorsalis pedis and posterior tibial pulses not palpable; popliteal pulses present. Weight 197 lbs. on bed scale. *Subjective data:* "I can't breathe—it must be my heart again."

Neurological

A 26 year old female was involved in an auto accident in which she had been pinned behind the steering wheel.

Immediately upon admission to the ICU, the following data were obtained:
a. Respiratory Status:
   —Breathing spontaneously with labored R at a rate of 40/min.
   —Breath sounds decreased on right side.
   —Oropharynx clear.
   —Nasotracheal tube in place.
b. Cardiovascular Status:
   —BP–126/84 mmHg.
   —Apical pulse–94/min.
   —Heart sounds within normal limits, no murmurs or rubs.
c. Neurological Assessment:
   —Responded to painful stimuli by decerebrate posturing of the right extremities.
   —No spontaneous movement on the left.
   —No seizure activity.
   —Pupils–Left–3mm and reactive; Right–7mm and nonreactive.
   —Gag reflex absent.
   —Blink reflex present on right; absent on left.
   —Blood draining from right ear.

Multi-system

An 18 year old caucasian male was admitted to the hospital after being involved in a motorcycle accident. His girlfriend, riding with him, was killed instantly. The initial diagnosis included a right pneumothorax with fractured ribs, a fractured pelvis, a compound fracture of the right femur, and multiple facial lacerations.

On admission to the emergency room, the nurse reviewed the vital signs recorded by the emergency medical technicians and obtained the following:
a. BP 110/70 mmHg, radial pulse–90/min regular, R 24/min labored, no chest expansion noted on right side. No breath sounds hear on right side. Breath sounds noted on left.
b. Abdomen was distended and rigid.
c. Right thigh was swollen.
d. Mental status–belligerent and agitated. Oriented to time, place, and person. An ethanol odor was noted on the patient's breath.
e. Multiple facial and scalp lacerations present; no drainage from ears or nose. Pupils equal and reactive to light.
f. N/G tube inserted–200cc light brown fluid returned.
g. Foley catheter inserted–400cc obtained–urine clear.
h. CVP–4 cm H_2O.

The patient had rambling speech, complaining of pain in stomach and right leg.

Renal

A 40 year old industrial accident victim is admitted to the critical care unit from the operating room after repair of his lacerated right femoral artery.

Upon admission, the nurse immediately assessed the patient's overall appearance and noted that he was responsive but drowsy; color was pale; reponded to various stimuli; had purposeful movement of extremities and was breathing adequately. His dressing was dry. He had whole blood and an IV of Lactated Ringer's solution infusing through separate IV sites. After initiating cardiac monitoring the nurse began a total patient assessment and systematically made the following observations:
a. Cardiovascular system— T 98°F orally, P 96/min, BP 124/86 mmHg (as compared to BP of 60/30 in the ER), no neck vein distention, heart sounds normal, cardiac rhythm–sinus; hands and feet cool with slow capillary filling in nailbeds; right dorsalis pedis and posterior tibial pulses faintly palpable and clearly audible per ultrasound monitor; left pedal pulses palpable; right foot cooler than left; right leg dressing dry.

Supporting Standards	Examples of Implementation	
	Respiratory	*Cardiovascular*

Neurological	Multi-system	Renal
d. Temperature: (Rectal) 101.2°F.	He cursed the driver of the car "for messing up my bike."	IV of Ringer's lactate infusing at 100cc/hr.

Neurological

d. Temperature: (Rectal) 101.2°F.
e. Evidence of associated injury.
   —Head—severe ecchymosis and swelling of right eye. Soft tissue swelling in right frontal area with small scalp laceration.
   —Neck—supple, carotids full bilaterally.
   —Abdomen—soft. Absence of bowel sounds.
   —Extremities—no apparent fractures.
   —Pulses palpable bilaterally.
f. Urine clear from indwelling catheter.

Multi-system

He cursed the driver of the car "for messing up my bike."

When he was admitted to the ICU, the critical care nurse immediately reassessed the patient's status to determine if changes had occurred.

Renal

IV of Ringer's lactate infusing at 100cc/hr.
b. Respiratory system—R 24/min and of normal depth, lungs clear to auscultation. No abnormal findings. O_2 at 4 L/min per prongs.
c. Neuromuscular system—patient verbalized but was lethargic; responded appropriately to stimuli; moved all extremities purposefully; demonstrated intact deep tendon reflexes.
d. Renal system—urinary catheter draining approximately 40cc/hr with no gross blood noted.
e. Gastrointestinal system—the patient has no difficulty swallowing; bowel sounds hypoactive; abdomen soft, nasogastric tube patent, draining bile.
f. Integumentary system—the patient's skin of normal turgor and intact with many bruises on his trunk and right flank.

The nurse noted the x-rays of the kidney, ureters, and bladder. These had been interpreted as within normal limits. The urinalysis was normal.

Serum chemistry values were: Na^+—141 mEq/L; K^+—4.8 mEq/L; Cl 104 mEq/L; BUN 19 mg/100 ml; and Creatinine 1.0 mg/100 ml.

Supporting Standards	*Examples of Implementation*	
	Respiratory	*Cardiovascular*
The critical care nurse shall collect subjective and objective data within a time period which reflects the gravity of the patient's problems/needs.	Because the patient's symptoms indicated a serious situation, the nurse gathered only the essential information within the initial 10 min period. After the patient's condition had stabilized to some degree, the nurse systematically proceeded with a thorough head to toe examination.	Because the patient was so short of breath, the nurse asked the patient to alert her if his breathing became more labored, explained that he would be receiving some medications through his IV to ease his breathing, asked briefly about allergies and the patient said "only allergy known is to shellfish." The nurse encouraged the patient to remain calm and reassured him that nurses would be with him until his breathing improved. This initial assessment was completed in less than 15 min due to the patient's shortness of breath. Approximately 2 hrs later, when the patient had considerably less dyspnea, the nurse proceeded with a complete history.
The critical care nurse shall collect data in an organized, systematic fashion to ensure completeness of assessment and concise communication of findings.	The nurse caring for this patient found that using a head to toe method to gather physical findings facilitated inclusion of all parameters.	This nurse organized the data collection by using the assessment tool provided by the hospital to ensure completeness of examination and documentation of findings.

The critical care nurse shall utilize appropriate physical examination techniques.	The following aspects of physical examination of the respiratory system were included in examining this patient.
	Inspection:
	  —thoracic contour/ deformities
	  —slope of ribs
	  —use of accessory muscles
	  —respiratory rate
	  —respiratory rhythm
	  —depth and ease of respiration
	  —cyanosis (central/ peripheral)—Pallor
	Palpation:
	  —tenderness/pain
	  —fremitus
		Objective data were obtained by using the following skills: Cardiac rhythm identification was carried out utilizing multiple lead placement.
		Inspection:
		  —skin color
		  —presence/absence of edema
		  —respiratory rate/depth
		  —jugular venous distention
		  —chest wall pulsations
		Palpation:
		  —peripheral pulses
		  —PMI (Point of Maximum Intensity)
		  —chest expansion

Neurological	*Multi-system*	*Renal*
Due to the comatose state of the patient, the nurse planned to gather the objective data quickly, within 20 min and then learn more about the patient's history from her husband when he arrived 1 hour later.	Because the patient was very agitated, much information had to be gathered from the patient's mother soon after admission including the fact that the patient had no known allergies. The nurse decided to defer the social/psychological data gathering until a time more appropriate for both patient and mother. During shift report, the nurse requested the next shift speak with family and friends.	Within the next 4 hrs the nurse continued with the exam: a. Endocrine system—the patient stated he had no family history of diabetes or other endocrine problems. b. Psychosocial system—the patient had an intact perceptual awareness of what was happening around him; he could talk about the accident and he seemed concerned about his wife and 4 children. He stated they were a very close, religious family and he asked to see his wife and a priest.
To ensure completeness, this nurse used a standard neurological check sheet as the basis of the exam, in addition to a body systems method.	Data were initially collected using the emergency room record form. The ICU nurse later compared the findings with those of the emergency room nurse and organized the assessment on the ICU flow sheet using a head to toe order.	This situation was aided by the initial use of a body system approach to assessment, with the subsequent formulation of a flow sheet to gather pertinent data at regular intervals. This flow sheet was modified to include all necessary parameters of this patient's care.

Objective data were obtained using the following physical examination approach:
Vital signs:
Level of Consciousness:
  —spontaneous behavior
  —response to stimulation
  —orientation
  —ability to follow commands
Speech and mental status:
Motor Function:
  —movements of extremities
  —grips
  —voluntary movements
  —involuntary movements
	Assessment of the abdomen involved the following techniques:
	Inspection:
	  —skin—scars, dilated veins, open wounds, rashes
	  —umbilicus—signs of inflammation, hernia
	  —contour of abdomen
	  —symmetry
	  —masses
	  —pulsations
	Auscultation:
	  —presence or absence of bowel sounds
	  —presence or absence of bruits
		The nurse would include the following aspects of the physical examination of the Renal System as part of the total assessment of this patient.
		Inspection:
		  —skin color
		  —skin integrity
		Palpation:
		  —tenderness
		Percussion:
		  —abdomen for ascites
		  —bladder for distention
		Observation of urine for:
		  —volume
		  —specific gravity

Supporting Standards	*Examples of Implementation*	
	Respiratory	*Cardiovascular*

Respiratory

Percussion:
— diaphragmatic excursion
— changes in density
Auscultation:
— quality and intensity of breath sounds
— presence and location of abnormal or adventitious sounds

Cardiovascular

Percussion:
— cardiac border
— diaphragmatic excursions
Auscultation:
— murmurs
— presence/absence of normal and adventitious breath sounds
— presence/absence of bruits
— normal/abnormal heart sounds

The critical care nurse shall demonstrate technical competency in gathering objective data.

Before assuming direct patient care responsibility the the nurse had satisfactorily demonstrated correct procedure for examination of the chest and technical competence in several diagnostic procedures, among which were:
— arterial puncture for blood gas sampling
— assembly of line equipment for continuous arterial pressure monitoring
— safe and accurate use of electronic devices for arterial pressure monitoring
— tracheal aspiration for culture and sensitivity

Before assuming direct patient care responsibility, this nurse had demonstrated competency in:
— application of multiple lead cardiac monitoring
— performing a 12-lead ECG
— assembling the flush system for pulmonary artery and arterial lines
— obtaining pulmonary artery and capillary wedge pressures
— obtaining cardiac output measurements
— physical examination techniques

Neurological	*Multi-system*	*Renal*

Sensation: Percussion/Palpation: —pH
Skin: —liver   —presence of blood
  —temperature   —spleen   —sugar, acetone
  —color   —gastric air   —color
  —moisture   —pain, masses   —odor
Pupil-size: —rigidity
  --response to light —kidney
Reflexes: —aorta
Cranial nerves: (As possible) —hernias

Because of the complexity of a neurological exam, this nurse followed a hospital-developed neurological evaluation sheet. However, each aspect of the exam had previously been satisfactorily demonstrated to the Clinical Specialist on the unit. Periodic in-service sessions were scheduled to assist the nurses in maintaining these technical skills. This month's session had included:

  —D.T.R.'s (Deep tendon reflexes)
  —pupil size and response
  —testing motor strength
  —testing cranial nerves

In addition to these physical examination techniques, the critical care nurse had satisfactorily demonstrated safe performance of the Intracranial Pressure Monitoring Procedure.

This nurse was currently orienting a new nurse to her unit and carefully explained the rationale for the steps used in examining this patient. It was stressed that auscultation is to be done prior to percussion and palpation to avoid altering auscultation findings in the abdominal exam.

This nurse had satisfactorily demonstrated competency to the Head Nurse of the unit in gathering the following data:

  —determination of jugular venous distention
  —ability to safely and accurately palpate and percuss the bladder
  —ability to palpate pulses in the feet and legs and to use ultrasonic monitor for auscultating pulses

Supporting Standards	*Examples of Implementation*	
	Respiratory	*Cardiovascular*
The critical care nurse shall demonstrate competency in communication skills.	Because of the patient's extreme dyspnea, the nurse asked only yes/no questions to minimize the patient's energy expenditure and oxygen demands. As the nurse explained what health team members were doing to and for the patient, nonverbal communication was emphasized, especially touch by holding the patient's hand and wiping her brow.	The patient's wife arrived to see her husband and was obviously upset about his hospitalization. The nurse discussed the patient's condition in terms his wife was able to understand. The nurse explained that the patient's breathing difficulties occurred because his heart was not beating as strongly as it should, and that he was receiving medication to help his heart beat more effectively. The nurse encouraged the wife to ask questions and express her concerns.
The critical care nurse shall gather pertinent physical, social, psychological, and spiritual data from the patient, significant others, and other health team members.	Since the nurse was unable to review the chart because the resident was writing an admission note, a summary of the patient's immediate history was obtained from the respiratory therapist who had been with the patient in the emergency room.	Although the nurse obtained much information from the patient, the wife was interviewed to determine other information pertinent to his care. The wife described her husband as a person who "is always working" and that he had been working long hours to get his new business going. She stated that he rarely complained of not feeling well. She expressed concern over financial problems while the patient was hospitalized.

Neurological	Multi-system	Renal
The nurse answered family questions in a manner that reflected interest in the patient and family members as individuals. The husband was allowed the opportunity to verbalize his fears and feelings of helplessness in a nearby lounge which provided a calm quiet environment. There, gathering data about the patient continued by using a non-threatening approach, open-ended questions, and good listening skills.	In order to obtain more data concerning drinking habits, the nurse applied the principles of crisis theory in communication with the family.	In communicating with the patient, a major area to be explored was his history concerning renal function. During the immediate post-operative period, however, the nurse realized that the patient was still groggy and, therefore, limited questions to the essential information; had the patient ever been told he had kidney problems; had he ever had a "strep infection," diabetes, or kidney stones; had he ever noticed blood in his urine, flank pain?

The nurse interviewed the husband and the parents regarding past medical and social history.
—Medical History: "Good health all her life"
—no significant cardiac or pulmonary problems
—no history of seizures or other neurological problems
—no medications. No allergies
—no prescribed diet restrictions
—one uncomplicated pregnancy
Social History:
—no substance abuse
—married four years
—English speaking
—education/occupation—High School graduate/Employed as a waitress
—patient/family experience with hospitalization, brain dysfunction—none
—religion—Mormon

On admission to the intensive care unit from the ER, the nurse noted the patient remained oriented to time, place, and person, but continued to be very agitated. He was able to tell the nurse where the pain was and that he was breathing comfortably. The mother explained that the patient had not been told about the death of his girlfriend. After talking with his mother the critical care nurse learned that he had never been in the hospital before. The nursing team therefore continually assessed his understanding of the explanations given him prior to treatments.

The nurse learned that the patient was a devout Roman Catholic and that the family was considering anointing the patient; the nurse referred a Roman Catholic chaplain to the family to assist in preparing the patient for news of his girlfriend's death.

Approximately two hours after admission to the unit, the nurse noted the patient's mental status was clearing. During each subsequent post-operative check the nurse continued to gather small amounts of information from the patient so as not to overly fatigue him. Assistance was sought from the emergency room notes and staff to determine the length of time the patient might have experienced hypoperfusion due to shock. The nurse also discussed the case with the surgeon during rounds.

Supporting Standards	*Examples of Implementation*	
	Respiratory	*Cardiovascular*
The critical care nurse shall collect pertinent data from clinic and hospital records.	Unable to elicit details of the previous hospitalization, the nurse requested the patient's old chart to gain information in providing more comprehensive care and preventing complications. Specifically, the nurse looked for any information omitted on the current history and physical. Numerous remarks were found about the extreme anxiety demonstrated by patient and spouse. The nurse also learned that a niece's visits had a very calming effect for both. She therefore copied the niece's name and phone number on to the current records for future use.	In reviewing the records of the patient's previous hospitalizations, the nurse determined that he was hospitalized for an acute anterior wall myocardial infarction one year ago. His recovery was uncomplicated, with no signs of congestive heart failure. Old records showed no other chronic diseases except for a seizure disorder which developed following a skull fracture and was well controlled with Dilantin. The patient had an abnormal glucose tolerance test during his last admission, but had normal fasting blood sugars. He had been discharged on an 1800 calorie, low cholesterol diet.
The critical care nurse shall utilize a current knowledge base in the process of data collection.	Representative clinical examples of this standard would soon be outdated because the critical care nursing knowledge base changes rapidly. The level and currency of the nurse's knowledge base can be measured via methods such as formal and informal testing.	Representative clinical examples of this standard would soon be outdated because the critical care nursing knowledge base changes rapidly. The level and currency of the knowledge base can be measured via methods such as formal and informal testing.
The critical care nurse shall collaborate with other health team members to collect and share data.	The nurse discussed the patient's respiratory status with the physician, respiratory therapist, and chest physical therapist, and the following decisions were made jointly: —arterial blood gases would be obtained 30 mins after intubation; then as needed following any major changes in vital signs and/or changes in ventilator settings. —the flow sheet attached to the ventilator would indicate all ventilator settings and subsequent results of arterial blood gases and vital signs.	The nurse noted the patient was showing a decreased systolic blood pressure and narrowing pulse pressures, increasing dyspnea and anxiety. He was producing an increased amount of pink sputum and had increased rales. The physician was notified of these findings and he inserted a pulmonary artery catheter and an arterial line. The nurse and the physician discussed these changes in the patient's condition and it was decided that: —the patient would receive 40 mg IV furosemide STAT.

Neurological

The nurse sent for old hospital/clinic records so that the data base might include any pre-existing problems which would influence the management of the head injured patient. Several routine physical exams, yearly pap reports, an uncomplicated obstetrical course, and two subsequent urinary tract infections were found. Also the patient's B negative blood type was clearly noted in the patient's current records.

Multi-system

Clinic records concerning yearly physical exams showed that he had had a functional heart murmur since infancy. No problems were identified in relation to the murmur. There had also been a previous fracture of the left wrist with no complications. His immunization record was not current for tetanus.

Renal

The patient's wife stated that he had been very healthy all his life and had required no hospital admissions. She also stated that his annual physicals at the clinic had been "normal." The nurse obtained the clinic records to collect data concerning his baseline renal function as a means of comparison during the current hospitalization.

Representative clinical examples of this standard would soon be outdated because the critical care nursing knowledge base changes rapidly. The level and currency of the knowledge base can be measured via methods such as formal and informal testing.

The nurse collaborated with the respiratory therapist and physician in collecting data with regard to a change in character of breath sounds and chest excursion. They agreed to:
—obtain arterial blood gases—STAT
—obtain vital signs and neurological signs every 30 min
—obtain sputum specimen for culture and sensitivity
The nurse and physician discussed the increased volume and decreased specific gravity of hourly urinary output.

Representative clinical examples of this standard would soon be outdated because the critical care nursing knowledge base changes rapidly. The level and currency of the knowledge base can be measured via methods such as formal and informal testing.

Observation—overstimulation. The nurse noted that the chaplain and social worker had been visiting the patient and family frequently. Patient's attitude: "I'm tired and need rest." The nurse called for a multi-disciplinary conference to pool information obtained from the interviews. The health team members then set up a visiting schedule and delineated areas of concern to be discussed with the patient by each member. It was decided that such sharing conferences would be held as necessary.

Representative clinical examples of this standard would soon be outdated because the critical care nursing knowledge base changes rapidly. The level and currency of the knowledge base can be measured via methods such as formal and informal testing.

Four hrs after admission to the unit the nurse noticed that the urinary output had decreased from 60 cc/hr to 30 cc/hr. The nurse recorded this on the patient's chart and alerted the physician.

Supporting Standards	Examples of Implementation	
	Respiratory	*Cardiovascular*
	—tracheal aspirate would be sent for culture and sensitivity immediately and thereafter according to unit policy.	—vital signs and pulmonary artery pressures would be monitored every 30 min, wedge pressure every hour, and cardiac output determinations every two hrs.
	—a baseline 12-lead EKG was to be obtained.	—the patient would have a urinary catheter inserted and urine output would be checked every hour.
		—breath sounds would be evaluated every hour.
		—the physician should be notified of urine output less than 30 cc/hr, and wedge pressure above 17 to evaluate for further diuretic therapy.
		—if urine output reached 1000 cc over the next 4 hrs, a potassium level would be needed.
The critical care nurse shall facilitate the availability of pertinent data to all health team members.	The nurse and the respiratory therapist documented all ventilator setting changes on the flow sheet. This allowed for proper coordination of lab values with ventilator settings and clinical status.	Flow sheets were used for continuous collection of data to record frequent vital signs, laboratory data, and treatments. The nurse not only included these routine parameters but also revised the flow sheet to accommodate pulmonary artery, pulmonary wedge, and cardiac output studies. The flow sheet was further revised to demonstrate relationships between therapies and recordings.
The critical care nurse shall revise the data base as new information is available.	Two hrs after admission, the patient manifested increased restlessness and agitation. Vital signs revealed: BP 170/100 mmHg ↑ by 20/10 HR 150/min ↑ by 25 RR 30 (ventilator rate 16/min)	The nurse reviewed the latest out-patient records and learned that the patient had been started on Digoxin during his last clinic appointment. In talking with his wife, the nurse learned that the patient had not been regularly taking his medication since he "felt fine," and,

Neurological	*Multi-system*	*Renal*

They planned to:
—obtain serum and urine osmolality—STAT
—obtain serum electro-lytes—STAT
—phone these results to the physician

This hospital had recently installed computer terminals for clinical record keeping. The nurse consulted with the charge nurse to ensure this information could be placed on the computer, and subsequently included all the observations in the format needed by the computer. To be certain of the content, a constant display of the data was arranged.

A permanent flow chart was used to provide on-the-spot current data to the health team. This sheet was specifically designed for use on this unit and allowed the nurse to assess the patient's condition quickly and make judgements concerning the monitoring frequency of the patient and/or the need for collaboration with other health team members. It also provided other health team members with concise, current information regarding the patient's condition.

The nurse recorded the designated observations on the unit's flow sheet. However, the policy of this hospital required making progress notes on all identified problems utilizing the problem oriented method of record keeping. This incorporated all aspects of data and was available for all health team members.

New Data:
—T (rectal) 103.5°F with excessive perspiration
—abdominal distention
—inability to close left eye completely
—mild tremors of both arms noted with stimulation of any type
—parents "blame the husband for the accident"

Observation—Altered Mental Status: While talking to the patient and his family about the accident, the nurse learned that he had several beers the night of the accident. The nurse also learned from his family that the patient seldom drank. The

Forty-eight hrs after admission the patient was oliguric and presented the following vital signs:
—BP 140/90 mmHg, up from 118/68
—P 108/min, from 96
—R 32/min, deep and rapid, from 21
—T 99°F (rectal)

Supporting Standards	*Examples of Implementation*	
	Respiratory	*Cardiovascular*
	ECG monitor showed sinus tachycardia with 4–6 multifocal premature ventricular contractions per min. The patient was questioned to determine if she were in pain, frightened, or experiencing dyspnea. The nurse examined the chest to note any changes. Arterial blood gases were obtained to rule out the possibility of hypoxia as the etiology of these changes.	therefore, did not have the prescription filled. The nurse then related this new information to the physician.
The critical care nurse shall document all pertinent data in the permanent record.	Before shift change, the nurse reviewed the charting to ensure that all subjective and objective data had been properly recorded.	The nurse requested that the unit secretary make sure all laboratory reports were posted correctly in the chart. Then the nurse transferred information from the flow sheet to designated forms in the chart.

Neurological	*Multi-system*	*Renal*
This new information was subsequently added to the existing data on the computer.	nurse made a notation on the record concerning the findings and updated the history section concerning alcohol habits.	He also appeared to be slightly disoriented, slow to respond to stimuli, lethargic, and had nonpurposeful movements of his extremities.
The nurse obtained a printout of the computer record to ensure that all data had been properly recorded. This printout was used during shift report to explain the problems identified.	In this hospital, the flow chart used by the nurse was considered part of the permanent record. In addition to including all objective data, there was a section for nursing notes which provided for recording of subjective data.	Progress notes were written on all identified problems utilizing a summary of the flow sheet data. A complete problem list was devised so that all professionals would address problems consistently.

COMPREHENSIVE STANDARD II: The identification of patient problems/needs and their priority shall be based upon collected data.

Supporting Standards	Examples of Implementation

The critical care nurse shall identify problems/needs based upon knowledge of the biological, physical, and behavioral sciences.

Respiratory

Problem: Difficulty communicating

Rationale: The patient was unable to talk due to the presence of the endotracheal tube preventing approximation of vocal cords and normal airflow between cords. Current physical state would make written communication difficult.

Cardiovascular

Problem: Congestive heart failure
—pulmonary congestion
—decreased oxygenation
—poor tissue perfusion

Rationale: The patient had an R rate of 36/min. Pulmonary artery pressure was 42/18 mmHg, wedge 17 mmHg, and an arterial lactate of 4.0. Chest x-ray showed cardiac enlargement and lung congestion.

The patient was exhibiting respiratory and cardiac symptoms of poor oxygenation, probably due to increased left ventricular failure and exudation of fluid into the alveoli. The fluid in the alveoli had greatly impaired oxygenation of tissues. Lack of oxygen delivery to the peripheral tissue had resulted in anaerobic metabolism with resultant metabolic acidosis and increased lactate levels.

Neurological

Problem: Increased intracranial pressure

Findings: Decerebrate posturing of extremities in response to painful stimuli. Pupils unequal, right 7mm and nonreactive, left 3 mm and reactive. BP 140/80 mmHg. P 100/min. R 35/min and labored. CAT Scan: skull series negative. Evidence of shifting of ventricles.

Assessment: Increased intracranial pressure related to cerebral contusion and edema. Possibility of intracranial hemorrhage with resulting hematoma, causing cerebral edema.

Multi-system

Problem: Pain in right leg after surgery for reduction of fractured right femur. Cast in place.

Observations:
—there was pain, dull in nature, associated with pressure.
—It was more severe in the proximal portion of the right leg, but had generalized to entire right leg.
—It was 2½ hrs post-op. Morphine sulfate was last given an hour prior to present onset of pain for an episode of sharp localized pain in the right femoral area.
—Pain should not have occurred this soon after narcotic administration.
　—It was a different type of pain than that for which the narcotic had previously been given.
　—The right foot was cooler to the touch than the left.
　—The right pedal pulses were decreased.
—Capillary filling was delayed on the right foot. There was marked swelling at either end of the cast.

Assessment: Arterial and venous impairment due to edema.

Renal

The nurse realized that the patient probably had impaired renal function as a result of renal ischemia suffered during the initial phases of his traumatic injury. The nurse also knew, from the previous total body assessments, that there were problems and potential problems that existed in relation to the cardiovascular system.

The patient had a BP of 144/90 mmHg and a slightly irregular P of 108. The increased BP, from the baseline of 124/86 mmHg was probably due to increased fluid volume and sodium retention as a result of oliguria but an increase in the reninangiotensin response to renal ischemia might also be a factor. The increased P from 96 and regular to 108 and slightly irregular was probably due to increased potassium levels but calcium levels would need to be assessed in the near future.

Supporting Standards	Examples of Implementation	
	Respiratory	*Cardiovascular*
The critical care nurse shall base all problems upon pertinent subjective and objective data.	*Problem:* Altered pulmonary status *Rationale:* Presence of infiltrate on examination, consultation on chest x-ray. Complaints of shortness of breath by patient.	*Problem:* History of seizure disorders *Rationale:* Patient stated he had been in an auto accident 5 years ago and had suffered a skull fracture. Over a period of time (approximately 4 months) he had experienced sporadic seizures which are now well controlled on Dilantin 100 mg. BID.
The critical care nurse shall hypothesize an etiologic basis of problems/needs, utilizing the collected data.	*Problem:* Cardiac dysrhythmia: sinus tachycardia with premature ventricular contractions *Rationale:* Cardiac monitor 12-lead ECG showed 1–2 multifocal premature ventricular contractions per min possibly related to myocardial hypoxia or underlying cardiac disease.	*Problem:* Financial difficulties *Rationale:* He owned his own business and would not have a steady income to support his 5 children while he was hospitalized.
The critical care nurse shall collaborate with the patient, significant others, and other health team members in identification of problems/needs.	The patient's husband identified her fear of the machine as a major problem. "She hates that tube and the breathing machine. Last time she thought she would die if she didn't stay awake to make sure the machine kept working."	The nurse asked the patient's wife if finances were a concern for them at this time. The wife indicated that they were but that the patient's brother would be of some help to them in this matter.
The critical care nurse shall establish the priority of problems/needs according to the actual/potential threat to the patient.	Priority of problems/needs: —altered pulmonary status —cardiac dysrhythmia —potential anxiety secondary to intubation, mechanical ventilation, and fear of death —difficulty communicating	The nurse immediately established that the patient's most severe problems were inadequate tissue perfusion and decreased oxygenation and their effects on various body systems.

Neurological

Problem: Adequate pulmonary ventilation

Findings: Blood gases reflect pCO_2 58 mmHg, pO_2 61 mmHg, pH 7.32 HCO, 2.75 mEq/L. Decreased breath sounds on right. Absence of gag and swallow reflexes.

Assessment: Inability to handle secretions, decreased level of consciousness, and right rib fractures contributing to ineffective ventilation.

Problem: Hyperthermia.

Findings: Temperature (rectal) 103.6°F with excessive perspiration.

Assessment: Probable hypothalamic involvement.

The patient's parents expressed great anger over the accident and it became apparent that an additional problem was emerging: difficulty in communicating among the patient's relatives.

On the basis of the collected physical and psychosocial data, the nurse identified the following problems which were immediately life-threatening and therefore the highest priorities:

Multi-system

Problem: Sensory alteration, inadequate and troubled sleep.

Rationale: The patient had been sleeping only at short intervals. Nightmares occurred daily. He had been in the ICU for 5 days. The patient tossed and turned calling out names whenever he slept.

Troubled sleep could be occurring in relation to:
—noise in the ICU
—anxiety about the ICU environment and his condition
—a high level of anxiety and nervousness that resulted from inadequate rest
—physical discomfort
—anxiety about status of girlfriend

Observation—Stabilization of mental status. The patient's altered mental status on admission had stabilized. He was now cooperative, oriented, and showed no signs of alcohol intoxication. His neurological signs had been stable. The nurses in the ICU discussed this with the physician and together they decided hourly neurological checks were no longer needed.

The initial assessment identified problems that needed solution immediately:
—pneumothorax that was compromising respirations and leading to hypoxia

Renal

Neuromuscular system: The patient was slightly disoriented and slow to respond to stimuli. He also had nonpurposeful movements of his extremties. The nurse contacted the nurse who had previously cared for the patient, and together they identified these changes in behavior as being a problem. The central nervous system and the muscular changes were probably a result of the effect of uremic toxins, metabolic waste products, and acidosis on the central nervous system.

Integumentary system—Pallor was probably due to overhydration and relative dilutional anemia. Bruises on trunk and right flank were still present. The nurse needed to be alert to skin color changes in the patient as his body attempted to use his skin as an organ of excretion.

The nurse asked the patient how he thought things were progressing. Frustrated with being sick, the patient angrily retorted that things were "just fine." The nurse decided that the patient perhaps had a need to ventilate his feelings, and allotted extra time to spend with him.

Having made a systematic assessment to determine the actual and potential problems, the nurse then listed the problems in order of priority as follows:

Supporting Standards	*Examples of Implementation*	
	Respiratory	*Cardiovascular*
The critical care nurse shall record identified problems/ needs.	The initial problem list was formulated according to the priority of patient problems/ needs. Subsequent problems were added to the list as they appeared and were identified.	*Existing problems:* —poor cardiac output —lung congestion —inadequate oxygenation —poor myocardial contractility —decreased tissue perfusion —history of seizure disorder (controlled) —need for education regarding disease, treatment, medication, & diet modification *Potential problems:* —cardiac/respiratory arrest —dysrhythmias —hypoxia induced disorientation —complications of immobility —seizures —prolonged absence from work

Neurological	*Multi-system*	*Renal*
—hyperthermia	—evaluation of the abdomen to rull out frank hemorrhage	—hyperkalemia
—inadequate pulmonary ventilation		—acidosis
—increased intracranial pressure	—reductions of the fractures	—oliguria
—inability to maintain fluid and electrolyte balance	—observation of the patient for head injury and its complications.	—arteriovenous shunt (patency and complications)
		—right thigh wound and repair of lacerated femoral artery
		—decreased bibasilar breath sounds
		—disorientation

Renal (cont.)

Potential problems:
—dysrhythmia
—volume overload
—hemorrhage
—infection–wound, and/or urinary tract
—clotting dysfunction
—anemia
—convulsions
—nutritional deficiencies
—gastrointestinal bleeding
—emotional maladjustment

Problem list:
—increased intracranial pressure
—inadequate pulmonary ventilation
—hyperthermia
—fluid and electrolyte imbalance

Although the history and physical data base may include a list of diagnoses, a separate list could be maintained with the nursing plan of care. Such a list could contain nursing problems as well as the patient's primary medical problems.

Problem List on Nursing Plan of Care:
April 12
    #1 Pneumothorax (resolved–April 14)
    #2 Fractured pelvis (reduced–April 12)
    #3 Fractured right femur (reduced–April 12)

April 13
    #4 Temporary problem— pain in right leg secondary to swelling beneath cast (cast bivalved–April 13)

April 14
    #5 Inadequate sleep

A list of the identified problems/needs was recorded on the permanent record. However, the list was also included in the nursing care plan and as each problem or need changed or was resolved, it ws also noted in the care plan.

COMPREHENSIVE STANDARD II: *(Continued)*

Supporting Standards	*Examples of Implementation*	
	Respiratory	*Cardiovascular*
The critical care nurse shall reassess problems/needs and their priority as the data base changes.	Forty-eight hours after admission to the critical care unit, the patient's status had stabilized. Short naps and decreased work of breathing had provided some rest and the patient was now able to communicate well using the writing pad. Although communication was not yet normal, it was satisfactory to the patient and health care team.	Admission work up showed blood glucose of 305 mg/100 ml, and urine sugar and acetone: 3+/negative. Hyperglycemia and glycosuria were added to the problem list.

Neurological

After 24 hours, the critical care nurse identified new problems:
1. Fluid and electrolyte imbalance due to excessive urinary output or second-stage stress response.
   —output average 400/500cc/h
   —specific gravity 1.001
   —serum sodium 170 mEq/L.
2. Seizure activity—focal seizure involving left side of face lasting 20 sec.
3. GI bleed—coffee ground gastric contents via nasogastric tube.

Multi-system

It had been 6 days since the patient was admitted to the ICU. His right lung was re-expanded and the chest tube had been discontinued. Vital signs had been stable and he had been afebrile. The morning ECG had been normal and chest x-ray essentially unchanged. Late in the evening, the patient suddenly became dyspneic and had sharp chest pain on the left side. Chest x-ray now showed an elevated right diaphragm. The priority at this time was to evaluate the pain (i.e., rule out pulmonary embolus) and initiate appropriate treatment.

Renal

The patient became more disoriented and did not seem to understand what the arteriovenous shunt was, or its purpose and he kept trying to pull it out. Thus, another need, to maintain the integrity of the AV shunt, was added to the list and included in the plan for care.

COMPREHENSIVE STANDARD III: An appropriate plan of nursing care shall be formulated.

Supporting Standards	Examples of Implementation	
	Respiratory	*Cardiovascular*
The critical care nurse shall devise a plan of care that reflects current knowledge of the biological, physical, and behavioral sciences.	To develop a plan of care that is based on current knowledge, the critical care nurse must avail him- or herself of ongoing learning opportunities to update his/her theory and practice base. (See Structure Standards, page 19.)	To develop a plan of care that is based on current knowledge, the critical care nurse must avail him- or herself of ongoing learning opportunities to update his/her theory and practice base. (See Structure Standards, page 19.)
The critical care nurse shall identify appropriate goals for each problem/need.	For two of the problems already identified, the nurse established the following goals: Altered pulmonary status —lungs clear on examination —optimal gas exchange and —pH level Cardiac dysrhythmias —normal sinus rhythm with a maximum of 2–3 premature ventricular contractions/min.	The patient's major problem was identified as congestive heart failure (CHF) due to low cardiac output from a poorly contracting myocardium. It was decided that the major emphasis of nursing care for the first 24 hrs was to increase the heart's effectiveness as a pump by minimizing the demands of the heart.
The critical care nurse shall determine nursing interventions for problems/needs.	For each problem, the nurse selected nursing interventions that could be done alone or with others' help. For example, to help the patient reach the goal of LUNGS CLEAR ON EXAMINATION, the following interventions were identified and written on the care plan: —examine chest and record findings every 4 hrs —chest x-ray as ordered and assess with physician daily —rectal temprature with P, R every 4 hrs —bronchial hygiene measures (percussion, vibration, postural drainage) every 4 hrs —ultrasonic nebulizer via ventilator for 15 min every 4 hrs per respiratory therapist —endotracheal suction every 2 hrs following respiratory therapy	To evaluate cardiac output, several assessment techniques were selected: —assess P, R, BP every hour —auscultate lungs every 2 hrs —record pulmonary artery reading every hour and alert physician if greater than 18 mmHg —note color and temp of extremities and presence/strength of peripheral pulses every 1–2 hrs —assess for changes in level of consciousness every 1–2 hrs —record accurate I & O; alert physician if urine output less than 30 cc for 2 consecutive hrs —weigh daily at 6 a.m. (with patient in slippers and pajamas) Interventions to maximize cardiac output include: —O_2 6L/min per nasal prongs

Neurological

To develop a plan of care that is based on current knowledge, the critical care nurse must avail him- or herself of ongoing learning opportunities to update his/her theory and practice base. (See Structure Standards, page 19.)

The patient-centered objective developed by the nurse was:

Absence of further deterioration of level of consciousness as evidenced by
—BP 100–140/50–80 mmHg
—P 70–100/min, regular
—T 98–100°F, rectally
—R 14–22, regular
—absence of seizures
—maintenance of current pupillary response

To achieve the goal of at least maintaining the patient's present neurological status, the nurse identified the following nursing interventions:
—assess P, R, BP every 15–30 min
—perform neurological checks every hour
—evaluate level of consciousness every hour
—elevate head of bed 30°
—maintain airway with endotracheal tube
—administer 30% O_2
—suction hourly and prn
—manually hyperventilate the patient prior to and immediately after suctioning
—hyperventilate on the ventilator (do not allow pCO_2 below 25 torr) OR hyperventilate with self-inflating bag prn for sustained elevation of intracranial pressure above 5 mmHg

Multi-system

To develop a plan of care that is based on current knowledge, the critical care nurse must avail him- or herself of ongoing learning opportunities to update his/her theory and practice base. (See Structure Standards, page 19.)

For the primary problem, right pneumothorax, the hoped for outcome was maintenance of adequate pulmonary functions evidenced by stable vital signs, satisfactory x-ray, pertinent laboratory tests within normal limits. The short term goals were prevention of pulmonary complications and removal of chest tube.

Utilizing a copy of the Standardized Care Plan for Pneumothorax as a guideline, the nurse outlined the care required specifically for this patient. The interventions regarding bronchial hygiene measures were modified so that they would apply specifically to this patient.

Renal

To develop a plan of care that is based on current knowledge, the critical care nurse must avail him- or herself of ongoing learning opportunities to update his/her theory and practice base. (See Structure Standards, page 19.)

For the problem of arteriovenous shunt, the goals were:
—to maintain patency of the arteriovenous shunt
—to prevent infection at the shunt site
—to stabilize the shunt
—to teach the patient and his family how to care for the shunt

In attempting to keep the potassium within normal range, the nurse took several actions:
—administered Kayexalate enemas as ordered to keep potassium in range of 4.0–5.5 mEq
—monitored potassium levels every shift
—observed for signs of hyper- and hypokalemia
—maintained potassium restriction of 40 mEq/day
—monitored I & O closely and recorded it every shift

Supporting Standards	Examples of Implementation ·	
	Respiratory	*Cardiovascular*
	—oral care every 1–2 hrs and prn —turn side–back–side every 2 hrs —check ventilator rate and assist control every hour —arterial blood gases daily and prn	—head of bed in 60° Fowler's position —bedrest with bedside commode for BMs —1200 cc fluid limit/24 hrs —2gm Na^+ diet —IV (liter D5/.2% NaCl) at 25 cc/hr —administer Fuorosemide 40 mg IV push every am and as ordered —administer Digoxin .25 mg orally every 9 am, check apical P —administer KCl 10 mEq/100 cc over 1 hour
The critical care nurse shall incorporate interventions that communicate acceptance of the patient's beliefs, culture, religion, and socio-economic background.	Through consultation with the patient and her husband, it was discovered that the patient was a night person. Arrangements were made for the patient to sleep as long as possible in the morning and be bathed in the evening.	One morning, the patient asked the nurse why everyone kept bothering him about fluids he drank in the hospital. After explaining the importance of an accurate I/O in relation to his condition, the nurse asked if he wanted to keep a record of what he drank. When he rejected the idea ("I am too tired"), the nurse accepted this—but noted on the Kardex that the topic should be explored further before discharge.
The critical care nurse shall develop the plan of care in collaboration with patient, significant others, and health team members.	While the patient was being mechanically ventilated, it was especially crucial for the nurse to communicate frequently with the respiratory therapist to set up the schedule for bronchial hygiene and nebulizer treatments. They decided that the nebulizer treatment would be given at 9–1–5–9–1–5 before percussion, vibration, and postural drainage. Suctioning would be carried out by the nurse after the postural drainage.	Because of the strict fluid restriction, the nurse needed to confer daily with the dietician to make sure that the patient's preferences were included on the tray in the appropriate amounts.

Neurological	Multi-system	Renal

—hypothermia to maintain T between 98–100°F
—restrict IV intake to 70 cc/hr of D5/.45% NaCl
—indwelling urinary catheter to gravity drainage
—nasogastric tube to intermittent suction/irrigation with normal saline to maintain patency

As the patient became more stable neurologically and more responsive, the nurse sensed that the patient was embarrassed at being bathed by the nurses. The nurse discussed this with the family, who asked to assist in patient care and in providing reorientation.

Because of the patient's reluctance to ask for pain medication as often as needed, the nurse indicated on the care plan that a pain medication, ordered on a 2–4 hr prn basis should be offered every 3 hrs and before chest tube removal.

The patient and his family were consulted about the normal patterns of activity for him as well as desired kind and number of visitors. A sign was posted on the door asking all visitors to check with the nurse before entering, so that he could sleep during his usual nap time of 4–6 p.m.

During the course of the evening shift, the nurse conferred with (1) the physician regarding maintenance levels of cranial intraventricular pressures and (2) the physical therapist regarding a plan for prevention of contractures and maintenance of muscle function by positioning, splinting, and appropriate exercises.

Since the physician had reported that the patient was going to surgery for stabilization of the fracture, the nurse asked one of the OR nurses to talk with the patient and family, and to help identify the patient's pre-op teaching needs.

The dietitian was contacted to talk with the patient to develop a diet which was within restrictions, but palatable. The physician, nurse, and hemodialysis staff developed plans to coordinate blood drawing, hemodialysis, medication administration, and physical care.

Supporting Standards	*Examples of Implementation*	
	Respiratory	*Cardiovascular*
The critical care nurse shall identify areas for education of the patient and significant others.	When the patient's husband asked what could have caused this problem to occur, the nurse decided that a topic for discussion later with the patient and her husband was the relationship between activity and respiratory status.	When talking with the patient about his medications and fluid and activity limitations prior to discharge, the nurse again discussed the relation of the fluid limit to the patient's heart failure episodes.
The critical care nurse shall organize the plan to reflect the priority of identified problems/needs.	Several problems had been identified by the nurse who prioritized the altered pulmonary status as the primary problem since that was the most threatening to the patient's well-being at this time.	CHF secondary to inadequate cardiac output was initially seen as the patient's major problem since resolution of this problem would correct several secondary problems: e.g., lung congestion, poor urinary output, decreased tissue perfusion, periodic confusion.
The critical care nurse shall revise the plan of care to reflect the patient's current status.	Initially the problem of inadequate pulmonary ventilation was of highest priority. Five days post-admission, the lungs were clear and the respiratory status stabilized. The patient was ready to be weaned from the ventilator. The major goal was thus changed to assisting the patient to adequately breathe without assistive devices.	After the patient's cardiac status improved sufficiently, the patient's major problem was identified as an inadequate knowledge base relative to management of CHF.

Neurological

Since the family had a number of questions about the equipment, particularly the computerized monitors, the nurse briefly explained their purpose and the meaning of the alarms that seemed to frighten the patient's family.

The priority problem initially identified was increased intracranial pressure, and the goal was to prevent further deterioration. As the patient's condition stabilized and the pressure lowered to normal limits, other problems took precedence:
—electrolyte imbalance
—hypovolemia
—persistent mental confusion

Over time, the nurse made the following observations:
—increased responsiveness to verbal stimuli
—presence of gag and swallow reflex
The assessment was that the patient had an increased ability to maintain an airway and the following interventions were discussed with the physician:
—remove the endotracheal tube
—suctioning every 2 hrs if patient not able to cough and deep breathe adequately on her own.

Multi-system

The physical therapist demonstrated and explained the patient's exercises to the nursing staff and family so that the staff and brother could monitor the exercises when the physical therapist was not available. This was reflected in the care plan.

Although the family was extremely anxious, the problem list reflected the fact that the pneumothorax was the most pressing problem. The nurse did give attention to allaying the family's anxiety while striving to stabilize the patient's respiratory status.

Five days post-reduction of the fractured right femur, the patient developed sinus tachycardia and a fever. A foul odor emanated from the cast. The cast was bivalved and pus and inflammation were observed at the operative site. The new problem and resultant nursing care implications were added to the nursing care plan and were given a high priority.

Renal

In evaluating the patient's readiness to learn, it was unrealistic to think that he would be able to learn how to care for his AV shunt at this time. Although it was still a goal to be met, action was deferred until the patient was more able to cope with it. Staff instructed the wife on shunt care for the immediate period.

A nursing plan of care was developed about 2 hrs after the patient's admission. This plan reflected a normally functioning renal system. Within the next 48 hrs, the care plan was revised several times to reflect a dysfunctioning renal system.

Problems: Hyperkalemia and Acidosis

Goal 1–A–to decrease the serum levels of potassium and elevate the arterial pH to normal

Goal 1–B–to prevent a rapid reoccurrence of high serum potassium levels

Evaluation: Hemodialysis is maintaining potassium and pH within normal range

New Goal 1–A–to maintain serum potassium and arterial pH within normal range

Supporting Standards	*Examples of Implementation*	
	Respiratory	*Cardiovascular*
The critical care nurse shall address all identified problems/needs in the plan.	Although the critical care nurse did not have time to complete nursing orders for all potential problems, some were listed for development once the patient's immediate crisis was over. Those listed were: —stress ulcers related to prolonged mechanical ventilation —ventilator dependence related to prolonged mechanical ventilation —muscle wasting/weakness related to immobility and impaired nutrition —compromised nutritional status	Although a complete plan of care was not developed immediately, the nurse listed all identified problems so they could be evaluated if they became acute. Other problems for the patient included several potential ones: dysrhythmias, pulmonary embolization, electrolyte imbalance.
The critical care nurse shall identify activities through which care is evaluated.	To evaluate the success of the nursing interventions for the respiratory problem, the nurse included the following interventions as part of the plan: —examine the chest —assess P, R, T —assess chest x-ray with physician	In monitoring the nursing care, the nurse observed the outcomes of the therapies: evaluated the patient's R, P, BP and urinary output, as well as any changes in strength of peripheral pulses; auscultated the lungs to check for rales; noted the changes in pulmonary artery pressures. Since the pulse had decreased from 120 to 108, the urine output was averaging 60 cc/hr, peripheral pulses were stronger, and the patient said he could breathe easier, the nurse assessed that improvement had occurred.
The critical care nurse shall communicate the plan to those involved in the patient's care.	Since so many individuals were involved in this patient's care, the nurse coordinated plans for a team conference and invited the following staff: the intern, resident, pharmacist, respiratory therapist, dietician, social worker, chaplain, the patient's evening and night nurse.	Since the nurses in this hospital were not permitted to chart in the patient's progress notes, the nurse alerted the physician to the patient's condition when the physician made rounds that afternoon.

Neurological

The problem/potential problem list to be addressed after the intracranial pressure and other related problems were brought under control included:
—possible stress ulcer
—possible infection
—possible corneal damage
—loss of bladder control
—inability to communicate
—possible extension contractures
—paralysis of left side
—family frustration, anger, and denial

Multi-system

Problem: Potential guilt feelings when informed about death of girlfriend in accident.

Plan: Ensure that the family understands the importance of stabilizing the patient physically before subjecting him to the stress of grief. Make all staff members aware of the decision to physically stabilize the patient before informing him of girlfriend's death.

Primary Outcome: Appropriate grief process is started.
   Immediate Goal
   —physical stabilization
   —exploration of grief

Renal

The critical care nurse identified several potential problems that the patient could encounter (e.g., dysrhythmias, volume overload, hemorrhage, infection). However, actions dealing with those problems would be deferred until all the priority problems were resolved, or until the potential problems became active problems.

The nurse evaluated the patient's status and the nursing care by monitoring the patient closely for the stabilization of vital signs. The return to a normal state of mentation was another parameter closely watched for, though taking longer to achieve.

During walking rounds at change of shift, all oncoming nurses listened to the primary nurse succinctly outline the patient's problems, current status, and the identified interventions. Questions were asked about his progress and one of the nurses suggested a different way to position the patient for greater skin integrity.

In accordance with the hospital's quality assurance program, the care given, as well as the patient's perceptions about the care were evaluated by the Quality Assurance Coordinator assigned to the unit. Although the care given followed hospital protocol, the patient expressed dissatisfaction with the meal routines. This information was communicated to his primary nurse who said the matter would be looked into.

The nurse communicated the plan of care to the other health team members via the care plan at the bedside and the progress notes in the permanent record. In addition, the family was kept informed since they were helping to monitor the patient's level of consciousness and were assisting in the reorientation process.

The patient was transferred from the emergency room to the intensive care unit with his chest tube in place. Within one hour, he was sent to the OR. While in surgery, the intensive care unit nurse talked with the ER nurse and formulated the plan of care.

This patient was discussed at the weekly patient care conference. At this time, a report on his status was presented and an updated plan was formulated.

Supporting Standards	Examples of Implementation	
	Respiratory	*Cardiovascular*
The critical care nurse shall record the plan of nursing care in the permanent record.	As new problems arose or old ones were resolved, the nurse made a SOAP note in the chart. Otherwise, at the end of each shift, a progress note on the patient's general condition was recorded.	Although not permitted to chart in the progress notes, the nurse made sure that the vital signs and information from the other interventions were completely recorded on the flow sheet.

Neurological	Multi-system	Renal
After initial assessment and therapeutic measures to control increased intracranial pressure were instituted, the written plan of care was developed.	The nursing plan of care was initiated and kept at the bedside. At the end of the shift, the nurse charted on the progress notes and, rather than again recording all the interventions identified, wrote under the Plan portion of the POMR note: "See plan of nursing care outlined on admission."	In addition to the periodic entries in the progress notes regarding the patient's status, the entire nursing Kardex was duplicated and placed in the patient's chart at discharge. This enabled the nurses, upon each of the patient's readmissions, to begin a plan of care that facilitated continuity and consistency by building on the previous admissions.

COMPREHENSIVE STANDARD IV: The plan of nursing care shall be implemented according to the priority of identified problems/ needs.

Supporting Standards	Examples of Implementation	
	Respiratory	*Cardiovascular*
The critical care nurse shall integrate current scientific knowledge with competency in psychomotor skills.	The nurse caring for this patient had practiced examination skills daily and compared these findings with those of others. In this way, skills were enhanced and the ability to accurately assess the effects of bronchial hygiene measures.	When repositioning the patient, the nurse placed him in a 45°, semi-supine position and supported his extremities and trunk in alignment using pillows. This modified position was necessary to minimize the decrease in PaO_2 resulting from the heart failure.
The critical care nurse shall implement care in an organized, yet humanistic manner.	The patient became fatigued and tense with minimal activity; therefore, the nurse spaced treatments to allow for rest periods, especially during the 11–7 shift.	At 49 years of age, the patient has had one myocardial infarction and now has congestive heart failure. He had been active with his work and family and was now quite ill. The nurse, recognizing the additional stresses for him, planned extra time for his care and to allow him to ventilate his feelings, and also arranged for a brother to visit for brief periods to update him on financial assistance measures being planned.
The critical care nurse shall provide care in such a way as to prevent complications and life-threatening situations.	Since the patient was being mechanically ventilated, the nurse wanted to prevent even minimal complications associated with this intervention. Nursing care was planned to reflect: —Prevention of airway obstruction through endotracheal suctioning and measures to reduce lung congestion. —Prevention of respiratory arrest through maintenance of mechanical ventilation with an oxygen source and self inflating bag at bedside in case of mechanical failure.	The nurse recognized that alterations in the cardiovascular system have a broad effect on the total body; therefore, care was planned to: —Prevent serious cardiac dysrhythmias by continuous cardiac monitoring and interventions as indicated. —Prevent electrolyte disorders by monitoring daily serum electrolytes and administering replacement therapy as ordered. —Minimize venous thrombosis and pulmonary embolism by implementing active leg exercises.

Neurological

The nurse monitored the intraventricular and arterial pressures and compared any changes in values with the overall patient status. It was recognized that data from electronic monitoring should not be used as the sole parameter for determining change in status because the electronic systems could be inaccurate.

By providing a quiet, relaxed environment and by talking to the patient and with the family, the critical care nurse reduced the intrusion of technology into the environment. It was also suggested the family speak to the patient about current family happenings.

Reducing the complications resulting from brain trauma was a primary focus for the care delivered to this patient. This included:
—Prevention of brain stem herniation by monitoring of intraventricular or intracranial pressure with use of hyperventilation and/or Mannitol and fluid restriction.
—Prevention of respiratory embarrassment and arrest by airway maintenance and bronchial hygiene.
—Control of electrolyte imbalance by evaluating serum electrolytes daily and appropriate replacement by administration of IV electrolytes.

Multi-system

The nurse milked the chest tubes every hour, as ordered by the patient's physician, carefully monitored the chest drainage, regulated the flow of the blood transfusion and calculated the patient's blood replacement balance.

The patient was to have his chest tube removed later in the morning. Since this could be a painful procedure, the nurse explained what would happen and that a small dose of analgesic would be administered. After gathering the necessary equipment, the nurse assisted in the removal of the chest tube, explaining each step of the process.

Because of the complex care needed by the patient with multi–system failure, the nurse planned the care to reflect:
—Prevention of necrosis and nerve damage by assessment of right leg circulation.
—Reducing occurrence of shock by monitoring hemodynamic status and administering fluids and drugs as ordered.
—Prevention of hemorrhage by observation of bleeding into cast and tissue swelling.

Renal

Since his serum potassium had elevated rapidly, the nurse closely monitored his cardiac rate and rhythm, measuring all intervals and observing for significant changes. It was determined that the necessary emergency equipment for treating dysrhythmias was available at the bedside.

This patient had intermittent periods of disorientation and restlessness. Since maintenance of shunt patency was imperative, the critical care nurse stabilized the cannula with a board and gauze wrap, restraining his shunt arm only after he hit the arm against the side rail and pulled on the cannula.

The nurse planned the care of the patient in order of priority to deal with potentially life-threatening situations. This included:
—Prevention of cardiac arrest by decreasing the patient's acidotic and hyperkalemic states.
—Prevention of hemorrhage by stabilizing and securing the arteriovenous shunt and observation of leg dressing for bleeding.
—Prevention of pulmonary edema by monitoring fluid balance.

Supporting Standards	Examples of Implementation	
	Respiratory	*Cardiovascular*
	—Maintenance of an accurate alarm system. —Prevention of life threatening dysrhythmias through continuous cardiac monitoring and lidocaine bolus at bedside.	—Prevent hypoxia and cardiac arrest through monitoring arterial blood gases every 12 hrs and administration of oxygen.
The critical care nurse shall implement the plan of nursing care in collaboration with the patient, significant others, and other health team members.	*Problem:* Possible fear of death. After meeting with the patient and her husband, the chaplain agreed to visit the patient each evening and to meet with her husband to discuss his concerns. When the patient began the weaning process, the nurse contracted with the patient's spouse to be present during the weaning and to provide encouragement and support.	The nurse contacted the appropriate health team members to implement the patient's care plan. The dietician discussed meal planning, with emphasis on restaurant dining within the prescribed dietary restrictions. The social worker arranged a meeting with the patient's wife to discuss possible sources of financial assistance.
The critical care nurse shall coordinate care delivered by health team members.	One person must coordinate patient care to ensure that efforts are not duplicated or therapies neglected. Since nurses have the most prolonged contact with the patient, family, or significant others and other members of the health team, nurses are in a prime position to coordinate patient care activities. Coordination responsibilities include: —Scheduling of therapeutic measures to ensure optimal effectiveness and patient rest/comfort. —Communication of all pertinent verbal and written data on an ongoing basis. —Conducting patient conferences with appropriate health team members for communication and problem solving. —Continuous updating of the nursing care plan.	One person must coordinate patient care to ensure that efforts are not duplicated or therapies neglected. Since nurses have the most prolonged contact with the patient, family or significant others, and other members of the health team, nurses are in a prime position to coordinate patient care activities. Coordination responsibilities include: —Scheduling of therapeutic measure to ensure optimal effectiveness and patient rest/comfort. —Communication of all pertinent verbal and written data on an ongoing basis. —Conducting patient conferences with appropriate health team members for communication and problem solving. —Continuous updating of the nursing care plan.

	Neurological	*Multi-system*	*Renal*

Neurological

—Prevention of hypovolemia from excessive urine output by monitoring of I and O, specific gravity, serum sodium and osmolarity, and appropriate replacement of IV fluids as ordered.

The nurse consulted with the following members of the health team to implement the plan of care:
—Physician—regarding medication, fluid therapy, level of intraventricular pressure.
—Physical Therapist—regarding prevention of contractures and maintenance of muscle function by positioning, splinting, and appropriate exercise.
—Biomedical Engineer—regarding arterial pressure and intraventricular pressure monitoring.

Multi-system

The nurse scheduled a multidisciplinary conference including the family to discuss the best approach for telling the patient about the death of his girlfriend.

Renal

A major part of the patient's care depended on hemodialysis therapy and maintaining dietary and fluid restrictions. The nurse needed to collaborate with the hemodialysis staff in terms of scheduling treatments for the patient, as well as to plan teaching for him and his family, and to meet the psychological needs that might arise as a result of the therapy.

One person must coordinate patient care to ensure that efforts are not duplicated or therapies neglected. Since nurses have the most prolonged contact with the patient, family or significant others, and other members of the health team, nurses are in a prime position to coordinate patient care activities. Coordination responsibilities include:
—Scheduling of therapeutic measures to ensure optimal effectiveness and patient rest/comfort.
—Communication of all pertinent verbal and written data on an ongoing basis.
—Conducting patient conferences with appropriate health team members for communication and problem solving.
—Continuous updating of the nursing care plan.

One person must coordinate patient care to ensure that efforts are not duplicated or therapies neglected. Since nurses have the most prolonged contact with the patient, family or significant others, and other members of the health team, nurses are in a prime position to coordinate patient care activities. Coordination responsibilities include:
—Scheduling of therapeutic measures to ensure optimal effectiveness and patient rest/comfort.
—Communication of all pertinent verbal and written data on an ongoing basis.
—Conducting patient conferences with appropriate health team members for communication and problem solving.
—Continuous updating of the nursing care plan.

One person must coordinate patient care to ensure that efforts are not duplicated or therapies neglected. Since nurses have the most prolonged contact with the patient, family or significant others, and other members of the health team, nurses are in a prime position to coordinate patient care activities. Coordination responsibilities include:
—Scheduling of therapeutic measures to ensure optimal effectiveness and patient rest/comfort.
—Communication of all pertinent verbal and written data on an ongoing basis.
—Conducting patient conferences with appropriate health team members for communication and problem solving.
—Continuous updating of the nursing care plan.

Supporting Standards	*Examples of Implementation*	
	Respiratory	*Cardiovascular*
The critical care nurse shall support and promote the patient's right to participate in his/her care.	The patient indicated she did not want her next chest physiotherapy treatment. Aware that the patient had experienced several procedures within the last 2 hrs and was especially fatigued, the nurse decided to omit the treatment. The rationale was that excessive fatigue would only nullify the benefit from the chest physiotherapy treatment.	Prior to beginning medication instruction, the nurse assessed the patient's knowledge of his drugs. He stated he was not interested in what the drug did. He would take the medication if someone could develop a schedule he could manage while at work. The nurse, the patient, and the physician worked together to develop a medication regimen.
The critical care nurse shall document interventions in the permanent records.	SAMPLE OF CHARTING: *Problem:* Altered pulmonary status *Intervention:* Percussion, vibration to lateral and posterior aspects right lower lobe, with patient in right side lying position with head of bed flat, followed by 20 min of postural drainage in same position. Large amount of thick rust colored secretions suctioned via endotracheal tube. Diffuse crackles over lower lung fields bilaterally.	SAMPLE OF CHARTING: S: "I don't feel like I am getting enough air." Denies chest pain. O: Blood pressure—150/90 mmHg; heart rate 100–120/min; pulmonary artery pressure 35–45/14–20 mmHg; wedge 15–21 mmHg. R 26–34 per min. pH 7.47; PCo_2 33; HCO_3 24; PaO_2 79. No sacral or pedal edema. Rales heard in both lung bases. S_3 still present. Weight 193 lbs. Furosemide 40mg IV given at 9:00 a.m. with 600cc urine output this shift. Started on Digoxin 0.25 mg orally every day. IV D_5W running well at 25cc/hr. A: Patient beginning to lose some excess fluid, but overt signs of congestive heart failure still remain. P: Monitor I and O and weights carefully to evaluate fluid balance. Plan daily hygiene procedures in short periods to prevent fatigue and increased heart rate. Observe for signs of digitalis intoxication and potassium loss after administration of diuretics.

Neurological

Although the patient was comatose and could not actively participate in her own care, her family showed considerable interest in her condition and her care. Her mother indicated she was interested in assisting with care but she was uncomfortable with bathing her daughter. The nurse suggested she comb and braid her daughter's hair daily.

TYPED INTO COMPUTER RECORDS

8:30 am—Intracranial pressure 17 torr. Decerebrate posture in response to pain. Right pupil reacts more slowly than left.

8:45 am—Intracranial pressure 19 torr. Ambued for 3 minutes. Intracranial pressure 15 torr.

9:00 am—Intracranial pressure 20 torr. Furosemide 40 mg IV given.

Multi-system

The nurse recognized the frustration experienced by the patient because he could not attend his girlfriend's funeral. To help him feel part of the preparation, the patient was assisted in calling the florist to order a floral arrangement.

RECORDED ON THE INTENSIVE CARE FLOW SHEET

1800 hr 12 April—sudden onset of sharp diffuse right sided chest pain; not relieved with change in position or breathing, no radiation. O_2 started at 8 l/min per mask for shortness of breath; physician called; blood to lab for CBC and arterial blood gases

Renal

While the nurse was cleansing and redressing the arteriovenous shunt sites, she became encouraged by the patient's questions and his interest in learning to care for the shunt. Eight days had passed since his injury and he now felt more alert and stronger; therefore, they agreed to begin the teaching of shunt care the next day.

SAMPLE OF CHARTING:

Problem: Arteriovenous shunt

S: No complaints of pain at site.

O: Bruit present; color bright red; insertion sites are slightly reddened; cleansed with hydrogen peroxide, betadine ointment and dry sterile dressing applied. Forearm positioned on board and rewrapped with gauze.

A: Shunt patent. Minimal inflammation at sites.

P: Continue routine inspection and dressing changes.

COMPREHENSIVE STANDARD V: The results of nursing care shall be continuously evaluated.

Supporting Standards	*Examples of Implementation*	
	Respiratory	*Cardiovascular*
The critical care nurse shall collect data for evaluation within an appropriate time interval after intervention.	The nurse reflected on the patient's response to therapy and on her own knowledge of the disease process. Utilizing this information, it was decided to re-examine the lungs and evaluate the chest x-ray with the physician after 12 hrs. In the interim 2 checks of vital signs would continue every 2–4 hrs or as indicated.	Immediately after administering an IV bolus of lidocaine for 10 premature ventricular contractions per min, the nurse evaluated the patient for change in rhythm and for untoward effects of lidocaine. Although the premature ventricular contractions were abolished and the blood pressure was stable, observation continued for recurrence of dysrhythmias.
The critical care nurse shall compare the patient's response to expected results.	Twelve hrs after beginning the bronchial hygiene regimen, the nurse examined the patient's response to the interventions. At this time, the patient's lungs remained congested, and her secretions were thick. The nurse had expected, upon auscultation, to find a decrease in secretions and crackles but this had not occurred.	Five days after admission to the coronary care unit, the nurse reviewed the patient's goals and nursing interventions. His weight had decreased 9 lb since admission. He felt he was able to breathe better. There was no neck vein distention. Heart rate was stable, 75–90/min, without serious dysrhythmias. Blood pressure was 120/74 mmHg. Crackles remained in lung bases. pO_2–90 at 2L O_2. The nurse noted the patient had the expected response to therapy for congestive heart failure. Digitalization, diuretics, and fluid restriction had decreased fluid retention.
The critical care nurse shall determine the relevance of the nursing interventions to the identified patient problem/need.	After 24 hrs had elapsed, the nurse reevaluated the patient's response. Secretions were mobilized and the lungs were clearing. This indicated to the nurse that the goal of clear lungs could be met through continued implementation of the plan.	Since the patient's status had improved in response to the therapeutic interventions for decreased oxygenation and poor cardiac output, the nurse determined that the goals were being met. However, patient instruction regarding knowledge of his illness and medications would have to be delayed until the patient demonstrated a readiness to learn.

Neurological	Multi-system	Renal
Several hours after the application of hypothermia, the temperature had reached the desired level of below 100.6°F.	At 2200 hrs, the nurse administered—Morphine sulfate 10 mg., subcutaneous for sharp incisional pain in lower abdomen.	The nurse evaluated the goal of maintaining the patency of the patient's arteriovenous shunt every 2 hrs. Although this time interval was usually adequate for maintenance of shunt patency, his shunt had clotted. Once the shunt was declotted, the nurse checked for patency hourly.
Laboratory reports from cultures of the sputum and urine would be reviewed when sent to the unit in 24–48 hrs.	At 2230 the patient was observed sleeping with no restlessness. Response to pain medication was satisfactory.	
Initially, the patient's T remained above 101°F rather than the desired level of 100.6°F. However, the nurse recognized that only a short time had elapsed since hypothermia was initiated and that the patient's T should drop after 2 hrs.	The day shift nurse expected an increase in BP with the fluid challenge and the patient responded accordingly. The nurse monitored the vital signs every 15 min to assess the patient's response, and then reverted to the physician's original order when the vital signs stabilized.	In response to measures to maintain shunt patency, the nurse expected the patient to have: —red blood in the tubing as opposed to dark-blackish blood, —no signs of clots or fibrous threads, and —evidence of a bruit. Upon examining the shunt, the nurse noted dark red blood in the tubing and was unable to auscultate a bruit, and became concerned that the shunt had again clotted.
Seventy-two hrs after admission to the unit, the patient's level of consciousness had improved. She was stable with no seizures; she had strong bilateral hand grasps in response to verbal stimuli; pupils were reactive to light and vital signs within desired limits. The nurse recognized that the expected goals were being attained.	The immediate goal of expansion of the right lung had been achieved as well as the short-term goal of chest tube removal. However, in 72 hrs the nurse noted signs of pulmonary embolism. In examining the nursing interventions related to preventing pulmonary complications, the nurse noted that measures to prevent embolism had not been identified.	With this patient's particular situation, the goal of maintaining shunt patency with inspections every 2 hrs was inadequate and another method would need to be devised.

Supporting Standards	Examples of Implementation	
	Respiratory	*Cardiovascular*
The critical care nurse shall base the evaluation on data from all pertinent sources.	In evaluating the treatment modalities for the problem of altered pulmonary status, the nurse gathered data from the physician, respiratory therapist, and chest physical therapist. Data from clinical evaluation were also gathered through physical assessment (general appearance, characteristics of tracheal aspirate, auscultation of chest, respiratory rate), and from laboratory data.	The nurse reviewed the patient's progress with the physician on morning rounds. The patient had shown significant improvement, the lab results reflected normalizing values, and the lungs were clear.
The critical care nurse shall collaborate with the patient, significant others, and health team members in the evaluation process.	The patient indicated that she was still dyspneic after suctioning, and frequently pointed to the endotracheal tube, wanting to be suctioned. Her husband, however, felt she was a little improved because she had better skin color. In discussing this with the physician, the nurse learned that the patient's lungs were clearer both by x-ray and by examination. They speculated that the basis for continued dyspnea was the patient's extreme anxiety in spite of the fact that she had improved clinically.	Five days after admission, the patient stated he felt much better and was breathing much more easily now. His wife reported that he was eating a little better, but that he complained of the diet being too bland.

Neurological

The nurse was especially concerned that data from the physician, physiotherapist, and comments from the family were incorporated into the evaluation.

In talking with the family, the nurse asked how they thought the patient was doing. They expressed great anxiety and fear of her dying. Since this was a perception not really supported by the patient's condition the nurse further explored their fears. Hearing them say the patient was acting so unlike herself enabled the nurse to identify the source of their concerns and provide positive information relevant to their concerns and the patient's actual status.

Multi-system

In reviewing the patient's nursing care, the head nurse consulted written records, interviewed the patient and his family, and then discussed the plan of care in a team conference. It was noted that all information obtained from these sources had been reflected in the written plan of care and in shift reports.

Problem–Fractured right femur.

Primary outcome—Full function of right leg.

Long term goal—Promote optimum healing.

Short-term goal–Ensure adequate nutritional intake at each meal. The nurse, concerned about the patient's inadequate dietary intake, talked with him about his eating. He stated that the food was not appetizing. The nurse asked if the dietician had been helpful. He stated that after he saw the dietician, the meals were better but that he was again being sent food he had not chosen.

Evaluation–The patient was not eating well due to food dislikes. The nurse communicated with the dietician to ensure that the patient's choices would be honored whenever possible.

Renal

In evaluating the care that was given to the patient, the nurse gathered objective data such as the results of diagnostic tests and physiological signs exhibited by the patient. However, the subjective and nonverbal data contributed by the patient and his family were just as valuable to the evaluation process. For example, in evaluating the goal of preventing infection at the arteriovenous shunt site, his verbalization of pain or tenderness in the extremity, or possibly his nonverbal behavior of lethargy could indicate the presence of an inflammatory response even before the nurse perceived inflammation through objective data.

The patient's statements about the condition of and sensation in his shunt extremity, as well as the family's response concerning the hemodialysis process, provided valuable data for the nurse in evaluating how specific goals were being met.

Supporting Standards	*Examples of Implementation*	
	Respiratory	*Cardiovascular*
The critical care nurse shall attempt to determine the cause of any significant differences between the patient's response and the expected response.	The patient's secretions remained thick and auscultation revealed that the lungs remained congested. Questioning whether the patient was sufficiently hydrated to allow for easy removal of secretions, the nurse reviewed the patient's I and O status, as well as the bronchial hygiene regime. Finding that the patient had only taken in 500cc in the last 12 hrs, the nurse hypothesized that: —The patient was not sufficiently hydrated to liquify secretions. —The frequency of bronchial hygiene measures was inadequate. —The humidification and bronchial hygiene measures were inadequately coordinated.	If there were no weight loss after administration of diuretics, the nurse would attempt to assess the cause: —Did the patient drink excess fluids after administration of diuretics? —Did a shock state exist decreasing renal blood flow? —Was the patient's cardiac status adequate to maintain a satisfactory cardiac output? —Were the recorded weights accurate? —Did the patient have excessive sodium intake?
The critical care nurse shall review the plan of care and revise it based on the evaluation results.	Having decided that high humidification would be helpful for mobilization of secretions, the nurse recommended the following interventions to the physician: —Ultrasonic nebulizer treatments for 15 mins/4 hrs for 2 days, then every 8 hrs for 2 days. —O_2 to be administered in conjunction with high humidity —Increase fluid intake to 1800 cc/24 hrs—ensure that patient achieves this intake.	If an adequate loss did not occur, the nurse and physician would discuss a more strict sodium and fluid intake, and increasing doses of diuretics.

Neurological

During the first 24 hrs, the patient's temperature continued to rise above 101°F when he was not on a hypothermia blanket. The nurse speculated this might be due to:
—neurological involvement (cerebral edema and increased intracranial pressure or hypothalamic lesion)
—infection.

Multi-system

The patient had become hypotensive and oliguric twice. In evaluating nursing notes and flow sheets, it was noted that no evaluation of mental status had been made for several hours prior to these two episodes.

Evaluation: The patient's behavior was not evaluated with the careful monitoring of the patient's fluid status and vital signs. Early signs of hypovolemia, related to changes in mental status, were not emphasized on the care plan.

Renal

The patient complained of pain in the shunt extremity. Upon checking the shunt site, the nurse found the extremity was edematous and discolored and blood was oozing at the insertion sites. The nurse had to make further assessments of the shunt to determine whether the shunt tubing had become displaced, a vessel had ruptured, or if the shunt was clotted. With the additional assessments completed and other health team members consulted, the nurse could then revise the plan of care related to the shunt.

The nurse needed to observe parameters indicative of neurological deterioration: level of consciousness, pupil signs, intracranial pressure and vital signs every 30 mins until stable. Since the patient's condition had remained stable for 4 hrs, the nurse changed the plan to assess the neurological signs every hour.

It was determined that the patient's hemodynamic state was not treated until he had become hypotensive and oliguric due to lack of emphasis in the care plan on early signs of hypovolemic shock. These specific concerns were subsequently addressed on the revised plan of care.

Since hourly monitoring of arteriovenous shunt flow had not been adequate to maintain patency, the physician decided to start a heparinized IV infusion pump. The nurse added this information to the nursing care plan.

Goal: Maintain the patency of the arteriovenous shunt.
—Monitor flow of heparinized solution hourly.
—Maintain secure connections between intravenous tubing, T-connector, and shunt.
—Evaluate for signs of generalized bleeding: e.g., hematuria, ecchymoses, melena.
—Request orders for coagulation studies in approximately 8 hrs.

Supporting Standards	*Examples of Implementation*

	Respiratory	*Cardiovascular*
The critical care nurse shall document evaluation findings in the permanent record.	**SAMPLE CHARTING:** Problem—Altered Pulmonary Status Goal—Lungs clear to examination O: Large amount of thick rust colored secretions suctioned per endotracheal tube. Diffuse crackles over lower posterior lung fields bilaterally. A: Secretions remain thick and difficult to clear despite bronchial hygiene measures. Plan: —Consult with physician regarding increasing frequency of ultrasonic nebulizer to every 4 hrs. Consult with physician regarding adequacy of systemic hydration. —Continue bronchial hygiene measures every 4 hrs. —Reevaluate status in 12 hrs. —Increase frequency of turning patient to every hour. (12 hrs later) O: Large amount watery rust colored secretions suctioned per endotracheal tube following bronchial hygiene measures. Right base of lungs clearer than left. A: Secretions being mobilized; lungs clearing. P: —Continue present bronchial hygiene regime. —Reassess efficacy in 24 hrs.	**SAMPLE CHARTING:** Problem—Low cardiac output causing decreased oxygenation and lung congestion. Goal—Increase arterial pO_2, mobilization of secretions, clear lungs. S: "I feel like I can breathe better today." O: PaO_2 now 90 mmHg. Crackles at bases. R 18–22 with tidal volume of 500–600cc. Producing ¼ cup watery sputum each shift. A: Able to cough, deep breathe, and bring up sputum better. Slightly improved respiratory status. Plan —pO_2 measurements on arterial blood gases done every 12 hrs —Auscultate for presence of normal lungs sounds every 2 hrs —Observe skin color for evidence of central and/or peripheral cyanosis —Evaluate R rate and quality every hour —Measure tidal volume every 8 hrs

Neurological

TYPED INTO COMPUTER RECORD:

Problem—Hyperthermia

Goal—Rectal T shall remain 100.6°F to normal limits.

Plan—Rectal temperature every 2 hrs. Acetaminophen Gr X for rectal T above 100.6°F. Hypothermia blanket for rectal T above 101°F. Examine chest, culture sputum, blood, and urine to determine if T elevation is neurological or infectious in origin.

Evaluation—(2 hrs after admission) Rectal temperature 101.4°F.

Assessment—Temperature control inadequate

Plan—Apply hypothermia blanket. Take temperature with a rectal probe to obtain continuous readings.

Evaluation—(4 hrs after admission) Rectal T 100°F

Assessment—T reduced to appropriate level.

Plan—Discontinue hypothermia blanket. Rectal T every hour.

Multi-system

RECORDED ON FLOW SHEET:

Problem—Fractured pelvis

Goal—Stable hemodynamic state after surgery.

Findings—BP was 84/50, HR 110, R 30; hands and feet cold with poor capillary filling. Urine O 25cc and 20cc the past 2 hrs.

Assessment—Low cardiac output possibly due to decreased volume status.

Plan
—Administer fluid challenge ordered by physician.
—Temporarily monitor vital signs and central venous pressure every 15 mins during fluid challenge.

Assessment—Vital signs and other parameters returned to normal and remained stable. Patient has slept very little the past 24 hrs.

Renal

SAMPLE CHARTING:

Problem—Arteriovenous shunt

Goal—To teach the patient and his family how to care for the shunt.
—Have the patient and his family describe how to care for the shunt.
—Nurse observes patient and his family perform shunt care on a mannequin for nurse to observe.
—Nurse observes patient and his family perform shunt care on the patient.
—Ask the patient and his family specific questions about shunt care.
—Give the patient and his family a paper and pencil test to evaluate their knowledge of shunt care.

Assessment—The cannula was securely in position with no sign of infection; however, the shunt was not patent. Therefore, the goal of maintaining patency was not achieved.

The patient had been able to describe the routine shunt care and to perform this on a mannequin. Therefore, certain criteria of this goal have been met.

REFERENCES   American Association of Neurosurgical Nurses. *Core Curriculum*. Chicago, IL: 1977.

Andreoli *et al.*, editors. *Comprehensive Cardiac Care*. St. Louis, MO: C. V. Mosby Co., 1980.

Bushnell, S. *Respiratory Intensive Care Nursing*. Boston, MA: Little, Brown & Co., 1973.

Harrington, J., and Brener, E. *Patient Care in Renal Failure*. Philadelphia, PA: W. B. Saunders Co., 1973.

Howe, J. *Patient Care in Neurosurgery*. Boston, MA: Little, Brown & Co., 1977.

Hurst, J. W.; Logue, R. B.; Schlant, R.; Wenger, N., editors. *The Heart*, 4th edition. New York: McGraw-Hill, 1979.

Lancaster, L. *The Patient With End-State Renal Disease*. New York: John Wiley & Sons, 1979. Chapter 2, pp. 1–60.

Meltzer, L.; Pinneo, R.; Kitchell, R. *Intensive Coronary Care: A Manual for Nurses*. Bowie, MD: Charles Press Publications, 1977.

Mitchell, P. *Concepts Basic to Nursing*, 2nd edition. New York: McGraw-Hill, 1977.

Nose, Y. *The Artificial Kidney*. St. Louis, MO: C. V. Mosby Co., 1969.

Oakes, A. *Critical Care Nursing of the Multi-Injured Patient*. Philadelphia, PA: W. B. Saunders Co., 1980.

Papper, S. *Clinical Nephrology*. Boston, MA: Little, Brown & Co., 1971.

Shapiro, B. A.; Harrison, R. A.; Trout, C. A. *Clinical Application of Respiratory Care*. Chicago, IL: Yearbook Publishers, 1975.

West, J. *Respiratory Physiology*. Baltimore, MD: Williams & Wilkins, 1974.

OUTCOME STANDARDS

Part II-C

VALUE
STATEMENT

The critical care nurse shall be cognizant of the intended results of care provided to the critically ill.

The preceding pages have addressed two types of standards for evaluating care of the critically ill. Structure standards are related to the environment in which care is delivered, as well as the credentials and requirements of personnel delivering care. Process standards are related to the nursing process or activities performed in the delivery of care. A third, and equally important, type of standard can be developed and relates to the end result of care delivery; this is referred to as an outcome standard. Although process and structure standards may be achieved, it is important to determine that the intended end result or outcome is also achieved. All three types of standards—structure, process, and outcome—are important and together provide a comprehensive approach to the evaluation of care delivered to the critically ill.

Outcome standards are not specifically identified in this document. They may be derived, however, from the process and structure standards identified in the preceding sections. The first step in developing outcome standards is to determine the purpose or intent of the process or structure standards. For example, examine the following process standard:

The critical care nurse shall provide care in such a way as to prevent complications and life-threatening situations.

The expected result or intent of this nursing activity is as follows:

Absence of life-threatening events

and

Absence of complications

These statements are examples of outcome standards and may be evaluated through an audit of the patient's health care record. Another example is illustrated using the following process standard:

The critical care nurse shall support and promote the patient's right to participate in his care.

Patient participation in various aspects of care is the expected result of this process standard, and the outcome might be stated as follows:

The patient participates in his care.

Or, if greater specificity is desired, the following outcome standards might be appropriate:

The patient monitors his own urine values

and

The patient correctly administers his daily insulin.

Evaluation of these outcomes may be achieved through record audit, direct observation of the patient, or patient interview.

Structure standards can also be converted into outcome standards. For example, examine the following structure standard:

Fire extinguishers shall be available within the critical care unit at all times and shall be inspected at least monthly with the inspection documented.

The outcome standards derived might include:

Fire extinguishers are available within the critical care unit at all times

and

Fire extinguishers are in operating condition.

Evaluation of these outcome standards might be accomplished through direct examination of the fire extinguisher. Finally, consider the following structure standard:

Additional knowledge and skills shall be acquired prior to assuming responsibility for the care of patient populations for which the nurse has not been prepared.

The actual intent of this standard relates to situations in which new patient populations are introduced into the critical care unit; in such instances, the intended outcome might be:

Critical care delivery is consistent with policies and procedures specific to the patient population.

Appropriate methods of evaluation could include record audit or direct observation of the nurse delivering care to the new population of patients.

Nurses involved in care of the critically ill are encouraged to develop outcome standards specific to their patient populations to be used in conjunction with the structure and process standards presented in this document. Integrating all three types of standards will provide the kind of comprehensive evaluation program required in critical care.

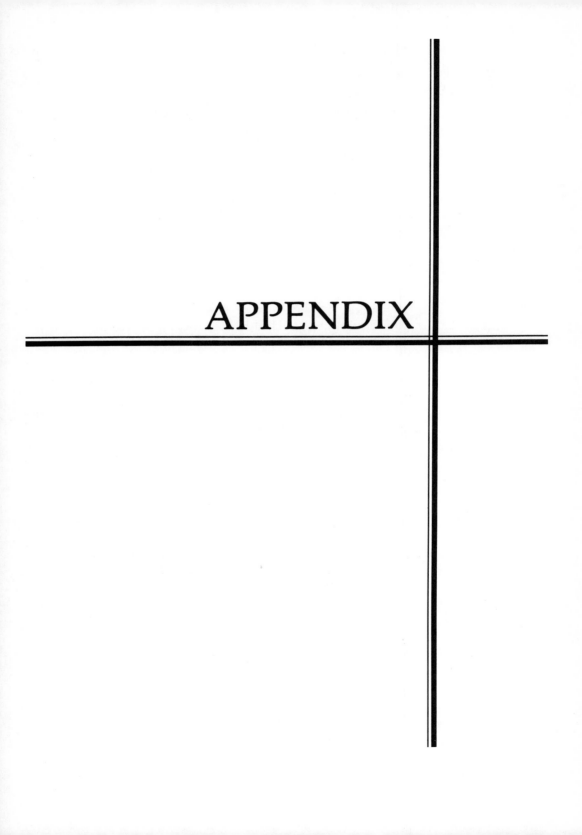

APPENDIX

STANDARDS STATEMENTS

Structure

I. THE CRITICAL CARE UNIT SHALL BE DESIGNED TO ENSURE A SAFE AND SUPPORTIVE ENVIRONMENT FOR CRITICALLY ILL PATIENTS AND FOR THE PERSONNEL WHO CARE FOR THEM.

The critical care nurse shall participate in the development of the philosophy of use, and in the designing and planning of any new or renovated critical care unit.

The critical care nurse shall be cognizant of various rules and/or regulations governing physical facilities for care of critically ill patients, such as those established by the:

—city
—state
—Department of Health, Education, and Welfare
—Joint Commission on Accreditation of Hospitals

The critical care nurse shall ensure the patient's privacy is protected without losing constant surveillance capability through the planning and designing of the critical care unit.

The critical care nurse shall ensure that the following components are considered in the planning and design of the unit:

—adequate space per patient bed, with consideration of potential equipment needs
—adequate illumination
—windows, clocks, calendars
—plumbing/sewage and sinks
—use of proper colors for walls, ceilings, and furnishings
—use of acoustic materials to minimize noise
—life support systems, including medical gases, suction outlets, and emergency power availability
—adequate space for support areas, including but not limited to:
—nursing station
—office space
—clean and soiled utility areas
—linen storage
—equipment storage
—medication room
—janitor's closet
—visitors' waiting area
—conference room
—staff lounge area
—nourishment station

—emergency equipment storage

—adequate ventilation and humidity/temperature control individualized for each patient room.

The critical care nurse shall ensure that a communication system within the unit provides for:

—routine patient care

—notifying appropriate personnel in emergencies

The critical care nurse shall ensure that the monitoring systems are appropriate to the needs of the patient population.

The critical care nurse shall be cognizant of the radiation hazards present in the critical care environment and shall strive to minimize untoward effects on patients, visitors and personnel.

II. THE CRITICAL CARE UNIT SHALL BE CONSTRUCTED, EQUIPPED, AND OPERATED IN A MANNER WHICH PROTECTS PATIENTS, VISITORS, AND PERSONNEL FROM ELECTRICAL HAZARDS.

The critical care unit construction, equipment, and operation shall comply with:

—applicable building codes

—state and/or federal occupational safety and health codes or standards

—current Life Safety Codes of the National Fire Protection Association

A member of the critical care nursing staff shall participate in the selection of new equipment which will be used in the critical care area. Instruction by the vendor in the use of new equipment shall be included as part of the purchase agreement.

All electrical equipment and/or electronic systems used within the critical care unit shall be inspected for reliable and safe performance. Such inspection shall:

—be performed by a qualified person

—occur prior to initial use, after repair, and thereafter, at least semiannually

—be documented

Resource persons shall be available to the critical care staff at all times to provide advice and/or service on electrical equipment and electronic systems.

Information regarding the use and care of all equipment shall be readily available to the critical care staff.

Written policies and procedures regarding electrical safety shall be established. Such policies and procedures shall include, but not be limited to:

—preventive maintenance programs

—general precautions in the care of patients requiring the use of electrically operated devices

—precautions in the care of patients who are particularly prone to electrical hazards, such as those with:

—debilitating conditions

—loss of skin resistance

—indwelling conductive catheters or cardiac leads

—severe electrolyte imbalance

—proper grounding

—restrictions on the use of extension cords and adapters

—prevention of overload to any electrical system

—inspection of electrical equipment and electronic systems

—disposition and servicing of malfunctioning equipment

—regulation and maintenance of appropriate temperature and humidity to prevent electrical hazard.

The critical care nurse shall demonstrate knowledge of and responsibility for implementation of an electrically safe environment and one which is consistent with established policy and procedure.

III. THE CRITICAL CARE UNIT SHALL BE CONSTRUCTED, EQUIPPED, AND OPERATED IN A MANNER WHICH PROTECTS PATIENTS, VISITORS, AND PERSONNEL FROM FIRE HAZARD.

The critical care unit construction, equipment, and operation shall comply with:

—applicable building codes

—fire prevention codes

—state and/or federal occupational safety and health codes or standards

—current Life Safety Codes of the National Fire Protection Association

A manually operated fire alarm system shall be available within the critical care unit.

Fire extinguishers shall be available within the critical care unit at all times and shall be:

—of the type required for the classes of fire anticipated in the critical care area

—located so as to be readily available when needed

—inspected at least monthly with the inspection documented.

A member of the Critical Care Committee shall be a member of the Hospital Safety Committee.

The Critical Care Committee shall ensure that policies and procedures which will minimize fire hazards to patients, visitors, and personnel are established and reviewed annually. Such policies and procedures shall include, but not be limited to:

—prevention of fire hazards in the presence of an oxygen enriched atmosphere
—use, storage, and transportation of gas cylinders
—fire drills
—fire extinguishing system
—evacuation plan
—reporting of fire safety policy violations

Fire drills shall be held at least quarterly for each shift, their occurrence documented and evaluated, and corrective action taken for any deficiency.

The critical care nurse shall demonstrate knowledge of and responsibility for implementation of all aspects of the fire safety program.

IV.   THE CRITICAL CARE UNIT SHALL HAVE ESSENTIAL EQUIPMENT AND SUPPLIES IMMEDIATELY AVAILABLE AT ALL TIMES.

The critical care nurse shall participate in establishing an inventory of necessary equipment and supplies for each unit that will:

—include routine as well as emergency equipment
—reflect the specific needs of the potential patient population
—be reviewed annually

The critical care nurse shall participate in establishing written policies and procedures for ordering, monitoring, and replacing equipment and supplies needed for each unit.

The critical care nurse shall ensure that equipment and supplies considered necessary during emergency situations shall:

—be centrally located and readily accessible, and
—have documented inspection at least daily by appropriate personnel.

The critical care nurse shall be responsible for ensuring the availability of necessary supplies and equipment before admission of a new patient.

Provision shall be made for replenishment of needed supplies on a twenty-four hour basis.

The critical care nurse shall demonstrate knowledge of and responsibility for obtaining necessary equipment and supplies.

V.   THE CRITICAL CARE UNIT SHALL HAVE A COMPREHENSIVE INFECTION CONTROL PROGRAM.

Written infection control policies and procedures specific to the unit shall be established and shall comply with any requirements directed by:

—national, state, and local agencies
—Hospital Infection Control Committee
—physical layout of the unit.

Written infection control policies and procedures shall address the prevention and control of infection among patients, personnel, and visitors. These shall include, but not be limited to:

—patient eligibility for admission, including requirements for equipment and personnel
—methods employed in the prevention of potential nosocomial infections
—storage, handling, and disposal of supplies, waste, and equipment
—control of traffic (hospital personnel and visitors) in the critical care unit and isolation areas
—inspection for outdated sterile items
—environmental disinfection and equipment sterilization
—nursing personnel assignment
—apparel worn by hospital personnel
—specific indications for isolation/precaution requirements in relation to potential or actual diagnosis
—responsibility and authority for initiating and enforcing infection control
—acceptable ventilation patterns, air exchange rates, air temperature and humidity.

The Critical Care Committee, in collaboration with the hospital Infection Control Committee, shall annually review and revise the unit's infection control policies and procedures.

The Critical Care Committee and the hospital Infection Control Committee shall devise an ongoing system for reporting, reviewing, and evaluating infections within the critical care unit.

The Critical Care Committee shall monitor all findings from any concurrent and retrospective patient care evaluations that relate to infection control activities within the critical care unit.

The quality of patient care shall be maintained regardless of the patient's need for isolation.

The critical care unit orientation shall include:

—introduction to the institution's infection control program

—individual responsibilities for prevention and control of infection.

Documented inservice education shall be provided concerning current infection control practices, pharmacologic interventions, and their nursing implications.

The critical care nurse shall demonstrate

—knowledge of the classifications of infectious conditions requiring isolation or precaution

—responsibility for implementation of infection control policies and procedures.

Infection control resources shall be readily available.

VI. THE CRITICAL CARE UNIT SHALL BE MANAGED IN A MANNER WHICH ENSURES THE DELIVERY OF SAFE AND EFFECTIVE CARE TO THE CRITICALLY ILL.

The critical care unit shall have a written philosophy and objectives which

—reflect the nursing service philosophy and objectives, and

—guide the nursing activities of the unit.

The operations of the unit shall conform to local, state, and federal laws.

The activities of the critical care unit shall be under the direction of a multidisciplinary committee, with appropriate representation from the medical and nursing staffs and other support services directly involved with the critically ill patient.

A policy and procedures manual shall be developed, annually reviewed, and approved by the Critical Care Committee, subject to approval by the hospital administration. Where appropriate, other non-nursing departments shall participate in the development of these policies and procedures. These shall include, but not be limited to:

—patient admission and discharge criteria

—use of standing orders

—decision-making roles of staff

—evaluation methods to determine effectiveness of the unit

—on-going requirements for continuing education of professional staff

—regulation of visitors

—regulations for traffic control

—safety practices for patients, staff, and visitors

—role of the unit in hospital disaster plans

—procedures for maintenance and repair of equipment

—patient care procedures, including specification of personnel to perform these procedures

—housekeeping procedures

—infection control measures

—list of necessary equipment for the unit

—electrical safety regulations

—fire safety regulations

—medication administration

—patient consultation and referral mechanisms

—discharge planning

—patient and family teaching

—documentation of the nursing care given

—maintenance of required records, reports, or statistical information

—scope of activity of volunteers or paid attendants

—initiation and termination of life-sustaining measures

The critical care unit budget shall be developed and administered by the medical and nursing directors.

VII. THE CRITICAL CARE UNIT SHALL HAVE APPROPRIATELY QUALIFIED STAFF TO PROVIDE CARE ON A TWENTY-FOUR HOUR BASIS.

Professional nursing staff shall possess the following qualifications

—current license

—documentation of the acquisition of a knowledge base with attendant psychomotor skills common to and requisite for the care of the critically ill

—willingness to participate in continuing education as indicated by past record

—current individual malpractice insurance.

Potential staff shall be interviewed by the critical care nurse manager for appropriateness of employment.

All professional nursing staff shall demonstrate knowledge of and responsibility for the implementation of the unit's policies and procedures.

There shall be sufficient professional nursing personnel to provide effective patient care. The nurse-patient ratio shall reflect recognition of the patient's acuity and required nursing care. Staffing patterns shall be reviewed regularly by the Critical Care Committee to ensure the delivery of safe care.

Unit staff shall participate in the development of staffing patterns. These patterns shall provide for:

—the flexibility to provide optimum patient care on a twenty-four-hour basis

—utilization of at least a 50% RN staff on each shift

—restriction of unlicensed personnel from delivering direct nursing care (except nursing students with an instructor present at all times)

—provisions for unit staff to function intermittently in a support role in other areas, but guaranteeing prompt return to their primary unit when needed

—contingency plans to ensure availability of qualified critical care nursing staff.

VIII. THE CRITICAL CARE NURSE SHALL BE COMPETENT AND CURRENT IN CRITICAL CARE NURSING.

Prior to assuming independent responsibility for patient care, the critical care nurse shall demonstrate possession of the knowledge base requisite for the care of the critically ill. This knowledge base shall include that content necessary for:

—collection and processing of data related to the physiological and psychosocial status of the critically ill person

—identification and determination of the priority of the patient's problems/needs

—development of a plan of nursing care

—implementation of the plan of nursing care

—evaluation of care delivered.

Prior to assuming independent responsibility for patient care, the critical care nurse shall demonstrate possession of psychomotor skills common to and requisite for care of the critically ill.

Prior to assuming independent responsibility for patient care, the critical care nurse shall demonstrate in supervised clinical practice the ability to integrate knowledge and psychomotor skills through applications of the nursing process and subsequent documentation.

Critical care nurses shall be responsible for seeking educational resources and creating learning experiences necessary for the achievement and maintenance of currency in their areas of practice. Such experiences may include, but are not limited to, the following:

—independent study

—nursing preceptorship

—inservice classes and grand rounds

—formal orientation

—academic classes

—seminars and symposiums
—rotating assignments under supervision
—affiliation with another institution for a specific learning objective
—tutoring by a nurse consultant
—patient rounds with members of other disciplines.

Additional knowledge and skills shall be acquired prior to assuming responsibility for the care of patient populations for which the nurse has not been prepared. Characteristics of a patient population to consider:
—disease modality
—treatment modality
—age of patients
—acuity

IX. **THE CRITICAL CARE NURSE'S PERFORMANCE APPRAISAL SHALL BE BASED UPON THE ROLES AND RESPONSIBILITIES IDENTIFIED IN THE JOB DESCRIPTION.**

Job descriptions shall be criterion-based, written and readily available for each classification of nursing personnel, and shall include:
—job title
—organizational relationships
—basic functions and responsibilities
—requirements and special skills needed
—expectations for continuing education

Nursing staff shall be evaluated at the end of the orientation period, at the end of the probationary period, and at least yearly thereafter, or as needed.

Nursing staff shall be evaluated by a variety of mechanisms. These mechanisms may include evaluation by:
—self
—supervisor
—peers

X. **THE CRITICAL CARE UNIT SHALL HAVE A WELL-DEFINED, ORGANIZED, WRITTEN PROGRAM TO EVALUATE CARE OF THE CRITICALLY ILL.**

The evaluation program shall reflect the following:
—current scientific knowledge
—professional and personal values.

The evaluation program shall include identified standards for care and criteria for achieving the stated standards.

Measurements needed to determine degree of standard and criteria attainment shall be obtained. Strengths and weaknesses shall be identified through interpretation of the measurements.

Possible courses of action based on the findings shall be identified and course(s) of action selected. Action(s) shall be taken.

Re-evaluation shall occur.

XI. CRITICAL CARE NURSING PRACTICE SHALL INCLUDE BOTH THE CONDUCT AND UTILIZATION OF CLINICAL RESEARCH.

The critical care nurse shall conduct and utilize research independently and/or in collaboration with others. Such activities should reflect:
—support and encouragement of nursing colleagues who are engaged in clinical research
—an awareness of one's strengths and limitations in various aspects of the research process
—current knowledge of clinical research in one's field of practice
—respect for a variety of types of research efforts, each of which can further the development of nursing knowledge.

The critical care nurse shall facilitate current and future clinical research through the consistent and accurate recording of data related to the patient's condition and nursing care provided. Such data should include, but not be limited to:
—physiological status
—psychosocial status

The critical care nurse shall implement changes in clinical practice only when the safety and effectiveness of the new practice have been established through an adequate research base and systematic investigation. Such changes must be accompanied by:
—a written policy change
—incorporation into an ongoing evaluation system or mechanism

The critical care nurse shall explore methods of sharing the findings of research efforts with nursing colleagues and with those from other disciplines.

The critical care nurse shall determine the potential hazards and benefits related to research involving subjects for whom she/he is responsible, including

—patients
—family or significant others
—personnel

The critical care nurse shall act to protect the rights of human subjects, including:

—the right to privacy and confidentiality
—the right to voluntary and informed consent without coercion
—the right to freedom from mental and emotional harm
—the right to know any potential harm or benefits related to participation in the research
—the right to refuse to participate or to withdraw from a study without fearing reprisal or jeopardizing care.

The critical care nurse shall be cognizant of and may participate in the mechanisms available to address violation of the rights of human subjects.

XII. THE CRITICAL CARE NURSE SHALL ENSURE THE DELIVERY OF SAFE NURSING CARE TO PATIENTS, BEING COGNIZANT OF THE VARIOUS "CAUSES OF ACTION" FOR WHICH THE NURSE MAY BE LIABLE.

Patients shall be fully advised in advance of all nursing and/or medical procedures to which they are subjected, signing a written informed consent when required.

Related causes of action:

Assault: An intentional act which places victim in apprehension of injury.

Battery: An intentional harmful or offensive touching without consent of victim.

Patients shall be allowed freedom of movement within their hospital room and are allowed to discharge themselves from the hospital.

Related causes of action:

False Imprisonment: An intentional act which results in victim's confinement within boundaries set by wrongful party.

Patients shall receive nursing care in accordance with good nursing practice and those policies specifically established by the hospital.

Related causes of action:

Negligence: A breach of a duty of due care which proximately causes injury to victim. Malpractice is the negligence of a professional. Required elements of negligence:

1. Duty of care (e.g., to perform nursing functions according to nursing policy manual);
2. Departure from duty (nurse fails to act in accordance with policy);
3. Damages resulted to the patient (patient suffers from monetary loss);
4. Causal connection between the departure and injury can be demonstrated (patient injured because nurse failed to adhere to nursing policy).

Patients shall be assured that any medical information will be shared only with health professionals treating the patient and that any other communication is restricted or occurs only with the consent of the patient.

Related causes of action:

Defamation: Invasion of victim's interest in reputation and good name by wrongful party intentionally communicating matter to third party (libel is defamation reduced to written or printed form; slander is oral defamation).

The patient's family members shall not be subjected to:
—incorrect information concerning the patient
—careless treatment of the patient

Related cause of action:

Infliction of Mental Distress: Intentional act results in subjecting victim to an emotional shock which is demonstrated by physical injury.

Patients shall be treated in a dignified manner, only those professionals directly involved in their care shall have access to their medical information, and this information will not be released or disclosed to others without their approval.

Related cause of action:

Invasion of Privacy: Using a victim's name or likeness for commercial use, intruding into the victim's private life, or disclosing private facts about the victim to the public.

Process

I. DATA SHALL BE COLLECTED CONTINUOUSLY ON ALL CRITICALLY ILL PATIENTS WHEREVER THEY MAY BE LOCATED.

The critical care nurse shall collect subjective and objective data to determine the gravity of the patient's problems/needs.

The critical care nurse shall collect subjective and objective data within a time period which reflects the gravity of the patient's problems/needs.

The critical care nurse shall collect data in an organized, systematic fashion in order to ensure completeness of assessment and concise communication of findings.

The critical care nurse shall utilize appropriate physical examination techniques.

The critical care nurse shall demonstrate technical competency in gathering objective data.

The critical care nurse shall demonstrate competency in communication skills.

The critical care nurse shall gather pertinent physical, social, psychological, and spiritual data from the patient, significant others, and other health team members.

The critical care nurse shall collect pertinent data from clinic and hospital records.

The critical care nurse shall utilize a current knowledge base in the process of data collection.

The critical care nurse shall collaborate with other health team members to collect and share data.

The critical care nurse shall facilitate the availability of pertinent data to all health team members.

The critical care nurse shall revise the data base as new information is available.

The critical care nurse shall document all pertinent data in the permanent record.

II. THE IDENTIFICATION OF PATIENT PROBLEMS/ NEEDS AND THEIR PRIORITY SHALL BE BASED UPON COLLECTED DATA.

The critical care nurse shall identify problems/needs based upon knowledge of the biological, physical, and behavioral sciences.

The critical care nurse shall base all problems upon pertinent subjective and objective data.

The critical care nurse shall hypothesize an etiologic basis of problems/needs, utilizing the collected data.

The critical care nurse shall collaborate with the patient, significant others, and other health team members in identification of problems/needs.

The critical care nurse shall establish the priority of problems/needs according to the actual/potential threat to the patient.

The critical care nurse shall record identified problems/needs.

The critical care nurse shall reassess problems/needs and their priority as the data base changes.

III. AN APPROPRIATE PLAN OF NURSING CARE SHALL BE FORMULATED.

The critical care nurse shall devise a plan of care which reflects current knowledge of the biological, physical, and behavioral sciences.

The critical care nurse shall identify appropriate goals for each problem/need.

The critical care nurse shall determine nursing interventions for problems/needs.

The critical care nurse shall incorporate interventions that communicate acceptance of the patient's beliefs, culture, religion, and socioeconomic background.

The critical care nurse shall develop the plan of care in collaboration with the patient, significant others, and other health team members.

The critical care nurse shall identify areas for education of the patient and significant others.

The critical care nurse shall organize the plan to reflect the priority of identified problems/needs.

The critical care nurse shall revise the plan of care to reflect the patient's current status.

The critical care nurse shall address all identified problems/needs in the plan.

The critical care nurse shall identify activities through which care is evaluated.

The critical care nurse shall communicate the plan to those involved in the patient's care.

The critical care nurse shall record the plan of nursing care in the permanent record.

IV. THE PLAN OF NURSING CARE SHALL BE IMPLEMENTED ACCORDING TO THE PRIORITY OF IDENTIFIED PROBLEMS/NEEDS.

The critical care nurse shall integrate current scientific knowledge with competency in psychomotor skills.

The critical care nurse shall implement care in an organized, yet humanistic manner.

The critical care nurse shall provide care in such a way as to prevent complications and life-threatening situations.

The critical care nurse shall implement the plan of nursing care in collaboration with the patient, significant others, and other health team members.

The critical care nurse shall coordinate care delivered by health team members.

The critical care nurse shall support and promote the patient's right to participate in his care.

The critical care nurse shall document interventions in the permanent records.

V. THE RESULTS OF NURSING CARE SHALL BE CONTINUOUSLY EVALUATED.

The critical care nurse shall collect data for evaluation within an appropriate time interval after intervention.

The critical care nurse shall compare the patient's response to expected results.

The critical care nurse shall determine the relevance of the nursing interventions to the identified patient problem/need.

The critical care nurse shall base the evaluation on data from all pertinent sources.

The critical care nurse shall collaborate with the patient, significant others, and other health team members in the evaluation process.

The critical care nurse shall attempt to determine the cause of any significant differences between the patient's response and the expected response.

The critical care nurse shall review the plan of care and revise based on the evaluation results.

The critical care nurse shall document evaluation findings in the permanent record.

OUTCOME

Examples supplied in Part II–C page 105.

Robert P. Benedetti, BS
Senior Chemical Engineer
National Fire Protection Assoc.
Boston, Massachusetts

Helen Benedikter, RN, BSN
Vice President Nursing
Long Beach Community Hospital
Long Beach, California

William Betts, MS, PE, CCE
Senior Clincal Engineer
University of Arizona
Health Sciences Center
Tucson, Arizona

Donald Billie, RN, PhD
Associate Professor, Dept. of Nursing
De Pauw University
Chicago, Illinois

Max Douglas Brown, JD
Staff Counsel
Michael Reese Hospital and
    Medical Center
Chicago, Illinois

Kathleen De Luca, RN, MS
Infection Control Nurse
Memorial Hospital
Hollywood, Florida

Carolyn Ehrlich, RN, MSN
Director of Nursing, Critical Care Ser.
Good Samaritan Hospital
Phoenix, Arizona

Paula Fleurant, RN, BS
Infection Control Nurse Coordinator
St. Vincent Hospital
Green Bay, Wisconsin

Rita Froelich, RN, MSN, CCRN
Administrator
Critical Care Services, Inc.
Chicago, Illinois

Eddie Hedrick, BS, MT (ASCP)
Epidemiologist
Morristown Memorial Hospital
Morristown, New Jersey

Harold Hirsh, MD, JD, FCLM
Clinical Assistant Professor of Medicine
Howard University College of Medicine
Washington, D.C.

Marguerite Kinney, RN, DNSc
Associate Professor
University of Alabama
Birmingham, Alabama

Norma Lang, RN, PhD, FAAN
Professor
University of Wisconsin
Milwaukee, Wisconsin

A. D. Lewis, PE
Deputy Director
Base Requirements and Utilization
Office of the Assistant Secretary
    of Defense (MRA & L)

Carole Lindeman, RN, PhD, FAAN
Dean, School of Nursing
University of Oregon Health
    Sciences Center
Portland, Oregon

Louise Mansfield, RN, BSc, MA
Professor, Emeritus
University of Washington
Seattle, Washington

Ida M. Martinson, RN, PhD, FAAN
Professor of Nursing
Director of Research
University of Minnesota
Minneapolis, Minnesota

Annalee Oakes, RN, MA, CCRN
Associate Professor
Seattle Pacific College
Seattle, Washington

Charles L. Rice, MD
Director, Intensive Care Unit
Michael Reese Hospital and
    Medical Center
Chicago, Illinois

John L. Ryan, FACHA, FAAHC
President, Ryan Advisors, Inc.
Health Services Consultants
Washington, D.C.

John P. Swope, MD
Captain (MC) USN
Director Program Support
Bureau of Medicine and Surgery
Department of the Navy
Washington, D.C.

CONTRIBUTORS
TO THE
PROCESS
STANDARDS

Karen L. Anderson, RN, BSN, MSN, CCRN
Clinical Specialist/Head Nurse–Coronary Care Unit
William S. Middleton Memorial Veterans
    Administration Hospital
Madison, Wisconsin

Charles L. Baer, RN, PhD
Professor and Department Chairperson
Medical-Surgical Nursing
School of Nursing
University of Oregon
Portland, Oregon

Pamela Jordan McCullough, RN, MS
Teacher-Practitioner/Assistant Professor
Rush Presbyterian St. Luke's Medical Center
Chicago, Illinois

Nancy C. Molter, RN, MN, CCRN
Major, ANC
Clinical Coordinator–Critical Care Units
Madigan Army Medical Center
Tacoma, Washington

Marilyn M. Ricci, RN, MS, CCRN
Clinical Nurse Specialist, Neurology/Neurosurgery
Barrow Neurological Institute of St. Joseph's Hospital
    and Medical Center
Phoenix, Arizona

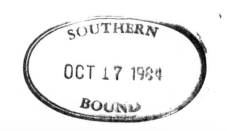